THE M BREAST

What You Should Know about GYNECOMASTIA

SREEKAR HARINATHA

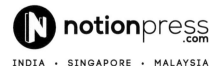

INDIA · SINGAPORE · MALAYSIA

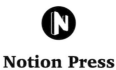

Notion Press

No. 8, 3rd Cross Street
CIT Colony, Mylapore
Chennai, Tamil Nadu – 600004

First Published by Notion Press 2020
Copyright © Sreekar Harinatha 2020
All Rights Reserved.

ISBN 978-1-64850-849-3

CONTENTS

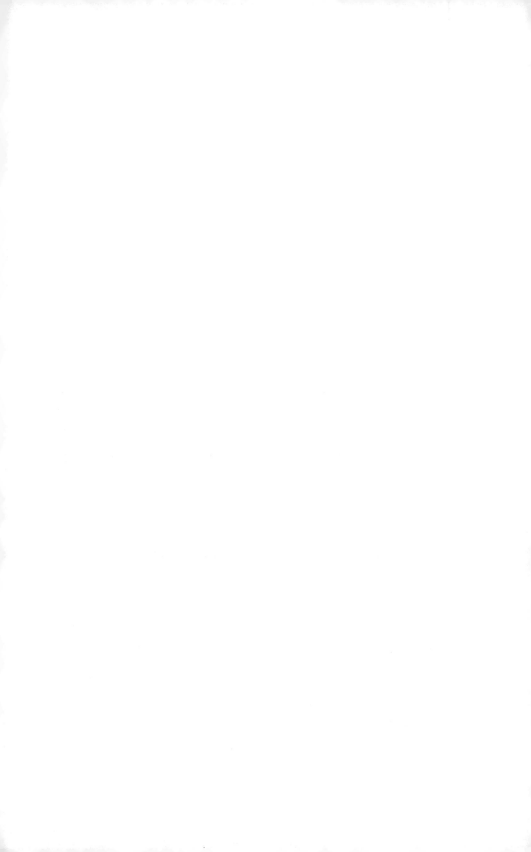

ACKNOWLEDGEMENT

To my dad, K Harinatha Reddy—I can barely find the words to express all the wisdom, love and support you've given me. You are my number one fan and critic and, for that, I am eternally grateful. In the process of putting this book together, I realised how true this gift of writing is for me. You've given me the power to believe in my passion and pursue my dreams. As the son of someone who has authored books in three languages, it is natural that a few dollops of the gift trickled down the gene pool my way, and I thank you for that. I could never have done this without the inspiration that you have always been. If I am blessed to live long enough, I hope I will be as good a father to Avyukt as you are, and always have been, to me. I love you, Dad!

To my mom, Padma Paradarami, who has always stuck with the family through the roller-coaster called life with unwavering dedication! You gave up the most important things in your life so that I could take on the most important things in mine. Mom, thanks for all the sacrifices you have made.

To my wife, Nithya Raghunath, who read the early drafts, gave me advice on the book and pushed me to finish the manuscript. You have been as crucial to this book getting done as I was. Thank you so much, dear.

To my son, Avyukt, you are the best thing to have happened in my life! I never knew parenthood would change me so much. Thanks for plastering a permanent smile on my face. You are the joy of my life.

To my brother, Sreeharsha Harinatha, you have always made me proud to be your big brother. I hope my books and writings are something that I've done in my adult life to make you proud too.

To my sister from another mother, Nikki, you are a vivid part of our lives. So let me just say an official thank you for being part of the family madness!

To Dr. Rajesh Powar, my mentor, who's skill and dedication were among the main reasons I got into plastic surgery in the first place!

Given that I'm poor at expressing my gratitude to people around me, I would try doing this here. It is also an acknowledgment of the positive influences of various people during different phases of my life.

To Vivek Akkera, Yashvanth Giriyappa, Sreedhar Gundappa, Kiran KJ, Sachin Dharwadkar, Ravi Thippeswamy, Shruti Mahadeviah, Hamsarani, Chethana, Srishail Chiniwalar, Satish Raikar, Pradeep JK, Sharath, Soundarya, Srikanth, Reeth, Supreeth, Vivek Saraf and the entire batch of JJMMC98 Gladiators from Davangere for helping me grow!

To Pawan Gandge, Sowrabh, Prashanth Bukka and Ramesh Sir from Bidar for the indelible memories.

To, Pradeep Baratakke, Pavan Kumar, Vishweshawariah Durgadmath and Sheela madam from Ranebennur for nurturing me.

To, Dr. VM Uppin, Dr. AS Godhi, Dr. Santosh Patil, Dr. Shirol SS, Ravi Reddy, Goutham Kamat, Prashanth Sajjan, Rama Velamuri, Ashwin Hebbar, Amol Mutkekar, Prashanth Puranik and Tejas Chiranjeevi from my time in Belgaum for all the timely nudges in the right direction.

To, Dr. Kiran Petkar, Dr. Rahul Shetty, Dr. Ashish Kumar Gupta, Dr. Kingsly Paul, Dr. Shashank Lamba, Dr. Arvind Lakshmanrao, Dr. Jewel Zacariah, Dr. Prema Dhanraj, Dr. Sandeep Dawre,

Dr. Naveen Kumar, Dr. Jeeth Jacob, Dr. Sowmya Khanna and the amazing nursing staff of plastic surgery department in Christian Medical College, Vellore for moulding into who I'am.

To, Dr. Vithal Malmande and Dr. Naveen Rao, from Apollo Hospitals, Bangalore for the wonderful experience.

To, Dr Ravikumar, my anesthetist, and my dedicated staff at Contura Clinic, Bangalore for being my daily sounding boards.

There are many more people I could thank, but time, space, modesty and my editor compel me to stop here!

FOREWORD

In the last couple of decades, the focus on male body image has been gradually increasing. Contrary to the common belief, it has been noted that men are equally, if not more affected by a negative body image than women. Vanity is no longer a prerogative of a woman. A deviation from the expected norm in the physical appearance can create a major upheaval in the self-esteem of a man especially during the growing years.

"All men are body conscious, if they say they're not, they're lying"

-Gilles Marini

The male breast has always been an enigma. It's function, form and aesthetics are replete with unanswered questions and controversies, both to the medical fraternity as well as the lay public. The aberrations in development and appearance of male breast are issues which have to be addressed with due importance. Such focussed issues need to be addressed through a well compiled treatise. Dr.Sreekar Harinatha has done more than justice to this in this book "The Male Breast"

The book has been well conceived, neatly compiled and extensively illustrated to cover the entire topic in an interesting and captivating format. The historical aspects, clinical scenario, assessment, medical surgical management, complications and post-operative care has been covered in a systematic manner. The photographic illustrations of various types and severity of afflictions of the male breast and the wide array of case series is impressive. The book covers the elaborate details of the issue at hand so as to provide a detailed understanding of the subject to surgeons and medical students. At the same time the presentation is so simple and lucid that even a common reader will be able to grasp it.

Gynaecomastia, which is the enlargement of the male breast is a frequently seen condition by a plastic surgeon. These patients are typically depressed, shy and introverted teenagers, rejected and dejected young adults, or frustrated middle-aged and older men. In fact, some of them have even undergone procedures by untrained and inadequately informed surgeons leaving them with scars and deformities which are as bad or even worse than the original problem. Surgeons treating these patients have to be abreast with the latest knowledge and honed with skills of the best techniques. This book will definitely serve as a guide to them.

I have known Dr.Sreekar Harinatha since his days as a Surgery Resident. The book reflects the discipline and meticulousness that he exhibited right from those days. It also showcases the vast experience he has gained in treating men who suffer from ailments related to the breast.

I feel blessed to be a part of two of the most noble professions of mankind-"Health Care" and "Teaching". Treating an ailing body and restoring it to normalcy is of course a very satisfying experience. What is even more fulfilling is nurturing a soul seeking knowledge. When you see your own student rising to newer heights and conquering newer horizons the sense of pride and jubilation one feels is difficult to describe. It is matter of great privilege for me to write the foreword to this excellent well-focused book "The Male Breast" by my illustrious student Dr. Sreekar Harinatha.

The book will be a valuable asset to a practising surgeon, a trainee surgeon and a medical student alike, as also to a reader with limited medical knowledge.

Professor (Dr.) Rajesh S. Powar,

MS, MCh, DNB

Professor & Head,

Department of Plastic Surgery,

KAHER's J.N.Medical College,

Belgaum, INDIA

BOY O' MINE

Boy o' mine, boy o' mine, this is my prayer for you,
This is my dream and my thought and my care for you:
Strong be the spirit which dwells in the breast of you,
Never may folly or shame get the best of you;
You shall be tempted in fancied security,
But make no choice that is stained with impurity.

Boy o' mine, boy o' mine, time shall command of you
Thought from the brain of you, work from the hand of you;
Voices of pleasure shall whisper and call to you;
Luring you far from the hard tasks that fall to you;
Then as you're meeting life's bitterest test of men,
God grant you strength to be true as the best of men.

Boy o' mine, boy o' mine, singing your way along,
Cling to your laughter and cheerfully play along;
Kind to your neighbour be, offer your hand to him,
You shall grow great as your heart shall expand to him;
But when for victory sweet you are fighting there,
Know that your record of life you are writing there.

Boy o' mine, boy o' mine, this is my prayer for you;

Never may shame pen one line of despair for you;

Never may conquest or glory mean all to you;

Cling to your honour whatever shall fall to you;

Rather than victory, rather than fame to you,

Choose to be true and let nothing bring shame to you.'

– Edgar Albert Guest

PREFACE

The male breast, known as gynecomastia, is a problem worldwide and is known by various names like man boobs, moobs, male chest enlargement, etc. It translates to 'female-like breasts' in a man. Though there are reports that up to 60 percent of men may be affected by it to a varying extent, the awareness in common men seems to be close to nil. It is estimated that 30 to 60 percent of boys exhibit gynecomastia during adolescence and that at least 30 to percent of these persist. A triple-peak in age-wise distribution is observed in the incidence of gynecomastia. The first peak is in the neonates, followed by puberty and lastly in old males. In each of these peaks, the cause is due to an altered hormonal status. Even in India, there is an increasing incidence of gynecomastia along with increasing awareness.

What causes gynecomastia is not fully known. Most of the causes fall into a category called Idiopathic Gynecomastia which means that gynecomastia occurs without any reason. The second category is called secondary gynecomastia wherein there is a known cause of breast enlargement like hormonal issues, chromosomal anomalies, Liver disorders, drug abuse, etc. This latter cause is found among a minority of the patients.

It is the aesthetic purpose that leads individuals to seek solutions for their annoying gynecomastia. Aesthetic satisfaction is a prominent concern for people who undergo surgery. So, the negligible surgical scar and the minimising of complications are crucial in this regard.

Whatever the reason, gynecomastia can definitely be treated. Such treatment not only improves the physical appearance of the individual, but also enhances the self-confidence and psyche. Whether you get it treated or no, the least you can do is know what it is all about and what your options are.

INTRODUCTION

When someone talks about a breast, the common mental picture one comes up with is a feminine figure, voluptuous and in all its angelic beauty. Admittedly, that figure is the most intricate and mystifying creation. But that same divinity probably despised this partiality among the two sexes and endowed many men with a similar bosom. This is the divine oversight that leads many men to explore the possible treatment for the illegitimate part of a male body.

The presence of breasts in men has been well-documented in history and mythology. Hermaphroditus is a famous Greek mythological character. He was born a son of Aphrodite and Hermes. A female spirit (Naiad), called Salmacis, fell in love with him and prayed to be united forever. God answered the prayer and merged their masculine and feminine forms and transformed them into a mixed androgynous form. Since then, Hermaphroditus became a symbol of androgyny and was portrayed in Greco-Roman art as a female figure with male genitals.

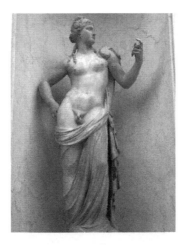

Hermaphroditus-The Greek symbol of Androgyny

Other religions and mythologies have vividly depicted male breasts, intersex and everything in between. The stories and myths range from 'Ardhanarisvara,' who was a culmination of Shiva and Shakti in Hindu mythology, to the shape shifting 'Jinn' or 'Shaitan' in Islamic folklore. In many tales and historical depictions, it was even an accepted norm for a man to have a slight bulge on his chest.

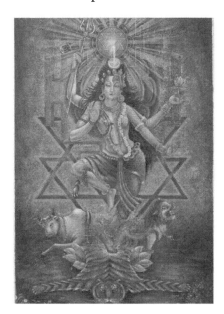 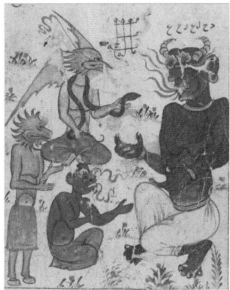

Ardhanarisvara and Jinn in mythology have been depicted to represent volatile sex forms

Tales apart, gynecomastia, or the male breast as it is commonly referred to, is a genuine issue. Gynecomastia is generally defined clinically as an enlargement of male breast tissue. It is characterised by the presence of a rubbery or firm mass extending diffusely and concentrically under the nipple and areola.

Most men with gynecomastia feel the presence of a firm to hard mass under their nipples during the puberty. Most notice it under their school uniforms. Many of them are subjected to jokes or ridicule, and some even suffer various psycho-social issues. Many students start wearing loose-fitting shirts during this period hoping that the gynecomastia gets less noticed. Many others try working out. I have seen many students in their high-schools, or in early their college years, working out endlessly in the gyms trying to burn the 'fat' under the nipples. They sometimes overwork enough to get disproportionately bulky chest muscles as compared to the rest of the body. Some extreme cases of steroid injections and unhealthy dietary supplement intake are not uncommon.

It's a common complaint from such a student's parent during the period that their son's self-confidence and outlook have drastically dimmed as he entered high school or college. Many attribute it to the academic stress or mental changes at puberty. It is further complicated by the fact that many such boys don't talk openly about the male breast with their parents which leaves parents guessing what suddenly went wrong with their kid. This can interfere with very important group/social activities including swimming, playing sports and participating in the gym.

One parent, in 2014, met me with their son who was studying in eleventh class. They were worried about the sudden drop in his grades and his low self-esteem. They had taken him to a psychiatrist too. The boy was on medication as he did not fully disclose the issue to the psychiatrist. Only later did he reveal gynecomastia to his father who, in turn, referred him to me. The boy had, in the last four years, been under severe psychological impact, apparently, as his friends poked fun at him for his breasts. He started wearing loose-fitting shirts on top of a male bra. Yes, you read that right—a male bra.

The male bra is a compression vest that is used following surgical correction for a few weeks so that the surgical swelling reduces faster. Many misguided boys wear it under their shirts to compress the breasts hoping that it would not show through their clothes and also hope that wearing it long enough would make the gland disappear.

Some others try bandaging—wherein they roll a tight and lengthy bandage or a cloth to compress the glands against their chest to hide it better. Some boys end up getting their skin damaged and even sustain rashes that have to be treated independently. The skin damage is due to the tightness and the subsequent skin irritation. The extent to which some men go to for correction of the breast is quite baffling; especially in these days where a simple Google search reveals that surgery is the straightforward option.

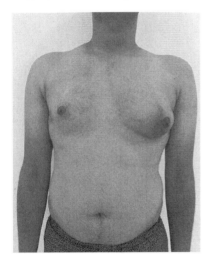 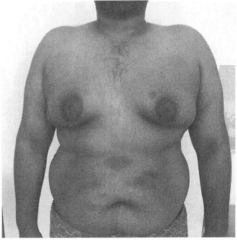

Men with skin irritation and eventual dermatitis following long-term use of the male bra

In August 2018, a very important and systematic meta-analysis was published on the psychological impact of gynecomastia and surgery. Meta-analysis is like an analysis of many research projects under one umbrella. In such studies, various other research patterns and results are analysed to give us a better and clearer understanding of the issue being researched on. This study was published in the 'Gland Surgery' journal by Martin Sollie from Denmark. They analysed over 500 research papers on the topic. They too noted that gynecomastia impacts the general health, functional capacity, social aspects, vitality and mental health of the individuals; all these were significantly and objectively improved once it was corrected by surgery. This is a seminal piece of information on the often-neglected psychological aspects of the male breast. There are many more detailed and meticulous trials and studies that second this conclusion.

Some of the known psychological effects of gynecomastia are:

- Reduced libido
- Body dissatisfaction
- Eating disorders
- Anxiety
- Low self-esteem
- Depression

Many studies have shown that the incidence of gynecomastia is highest during puberty. The percentages vary from 20 to 60 percent. Though this seems like a very high number, it does, however, give us an insight into the wide prevalence of male breasts. It's not as rare as one might think. There is also a wide difference in its occurrence among various races. Asians and Indians are perched right at the top of the pile, while Caucasians experience far lesser incidence of gynecomastia.

Now, it does seem strange that an issue that affects such a large populous is discussed so little among mainstream media and has so few books written on them. There is a glaring lacuna and knowledge-gap among men. This book endeavours to fill that gap as much as it can. As I go through, I would be discussing the various aspects of gynecomastia with a special emphasis on the treatment. So if you have gynecomastia, the least you can do is know what it is all about and what you can do about it.

Psychological Effects of Gynecomastia

1 DEPRESSION

2 LOW SELF-ESTEEM

3 ANXIETY

4 EATING DISORDERS

5 BODY DISSATISFACTION

6 REDUCED LIBIDO

www.gynecomastiabangalore.com

Chapter 1

WHAT IS MALE BREAST AND WHY DOES IT OCCUR

The Medical Definition: Gynecomastia is defined clinically as an enlargement of male breast tissue. It is characterised by the presence of a rubbery or firm mass extending diffusely and concentrically under the nipple and areola.

The Common Man's Definition: chest fat, male boobs, moobs, male breast, etc.

It's common in my practice to have a patient come in saying that he has a lot of chest fat and wants it sorted. Most of these people are usually quite fit and don't even have a lot of fat in their body to begin with. Many would have worked out endlessly only to notice that the chest bulge hasn't reduced. If anything, the 'chest fat' is now more prominent and protruding than it was when they were less fit. Many men, who do not research or take a medical opinion, finally attribute this to 'stubborn fat'. Only when a doctor examines and points out the differences in how the 'chest fat' feels as opposed to the fat elsewhere do they realise that it's something else. Some people feel crestfallen when confronted by the diagnosis.

In my practice, bodybuilders with gynecomastia are not unusual. I'm frequently visited by bodybuilders with gynecomastia. I vividly remember a bodybuilder who was aspiring to compete in an international bodybuilding competition. He was very muscular almost like Arnold Schwarzenegger. He had a nice set of eight-packs and huge biceps; but he also had two puffy nipples. He worked out so much to reduce the 'chest fat,' that his chest muscles were abnormally bulky even for his muscular physique. It was only when a trainer told him to get it checked that he came to me.

The 'Bodybuilder's Gynecomastia', as it is commonly referred to, is usually small (confined to the area just under the areola) and is a result of self-medicating with hormones and anabolic steroids to bulk up their muscles. They have very low percentages of body fat and are in good physical shape. These bodybuilders get gynecomastia following usage of self-prescribed (or gym trainer prescribed) medications, which disrupt the delicate hormonal balance. It is common for me to encounter men with six pack abs and well-built muscles presenting with gynecomastia.

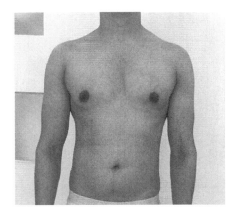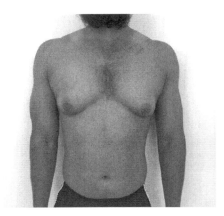

Bodybuilders' Gynecomastia

Some men do not explicitly take anabolic steroids. They may take 'protein supplements', prohormones and other seemingly harmless supplements available at health food stores or through the internet. The problem is that, many of the listed ingredients are not specific and these supplements may indeed have hormone-like qualities. The net-effect is that gynecomastia may develop most unexpectedly and, sometimes, very quickly. Once it has developed, there are no treatments for it other than surgery.

A study conducted by Blau M and Hazani R. ('Correction of gynecomastia in bodybuilders and patients with good physique,' published in the Plastic and Reconstructive Surgery journal in 2015) stresses the importance of direct removal of the glandular tissue over any other surgical technique when correcting gynecomastia in bodybuilders. They also advise that a novice surgeon is advised to proceed with cases that are less challenging and leave such cases to experienced surgeons. (*https://pubmed.ncbi.nlm.nih.gov/25626789/*)

Male breast reduction surgery for Bangalore (Bengaluru) bodybuilders is very similar to the standard procedure described elsewhere on this website. There are some significant differences, however.

1. Steroid-induced gynecomastia is solid, white and hard as compared to pubertal gynecomastia. There is very little peripheral fat in bodybuilders.

2. Liposuction is done more often to help re-distribute the skin across the chest than to remove the fat. The net-effect after healing is that of a very thin and uniform layer of skin and fat which is now draped over the large pec muscle, thereby providing the desired "muscular" appearance.

3. Anaesthesia for this surgery is provided by a separate anaesthesiologist.

4. A compression garment is provided and should be worn 24/7 for several weeks. A return to strenuous exercise should be deferred for several weeks as well, to allow for appropriate healing.

The results of gynecomastia surgery in bodybuilders are usually permanent, provided that additional illicit drugs are not used in the future. There is always a small amount of breast tissue deliberately left under the areola to prevent a crater deformity. Should additional drugs be taken in the future, it is that residual breast tissue that can possibly regrow again with hormonal supplements.

When a male breast is seen under a microscope, it contains what we call 'a benign proliferation of glandular male breast tissue'. Microscopically, the tissue is very similar to a female breast. But, of course, the tissue is different functionally in the sense that it does not produce milk. It means that it serves no function in males and is a vestigial and purposeless tissue.

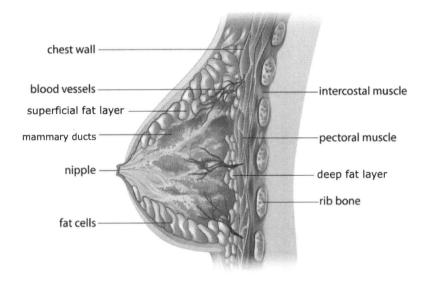

Breast structure is strikingly similar in males and females

During puberty, changes in the breast bud occur due to the hormonal influence and lead to transient enlargement of the breasts and it is, in fact, a very common occurrence. It becomes an issue when this enlargement either becomes too excessive or fails to regress in time. The psychological impact that can result during these very important, formative years can have long-lasting effects on the emotional and social development of the individual.

Male breast development occurs in a similar fashion to that of female breast development. At puberty, in the female, complex hormonal interplay results in the growth and maturation of the adult female breast.

Gynecomastia normally can occur during three phases of life.

The first occurs shortly after birth in both males and females. This is caused by the high levels of predominantly feminine hormones;

estradiol and progesterone produced by the mother during pregnancy, which stimulates the new-born breast tissue. It can persist for several weeks after birth.

Puberty is the second phase in which gynecomastia can occur physiologically. This again is due to the imbalance of hormones. It may be due to either decreased production of androgens (male hormones) or change in its ratio in relation to the female hormones.

The third age-range in which gynecomastia is frequently seen is during older age (over 60 years). Although the exact mechanisms by which this can occur are not fully clear, it may result from reduced male hormone production associated with ageing and other factors.

In early fetal (when the baby is still in the mother's womb) life, epithelial cells (cells on the skin's surface) that are destined to become areola also form the ducts. The ducts are the supply pipelines through which the mother's milk which is produced in the alveolar structures (the milk-producing part of the breast) are transported to the nipple. As the influence of the mother's hormones that are transferred to the baby while in the womb reduces, the breast development ceases. This process of multiplication and tissue-replication restarts when the hormonal balance is altered like in puberty. But, once the hormonal issues regress, the tissue also tends to reduce when it's not large enough. But, in many men, even after the hormonal influence ceases, the gland persists and leads to all the issues related to breast enlargement

In puberty, when the gland develops and gets noticeable, many complain of pain and tenderness which sometimes leads them to medical consultation. Evaluation under the guidance of a physician can be performed as needed to rule out other conditions that can result in hormonal imbalance affecting the breast. Although it is reasonable to simply observe patients who present with gynecomastia even until the age of 16 or 18, when social behaviours begin to become negatively affected by the condition, it is recommended to proceed with surgical correction nonetheless in many cases.

But most patients, however, overlook and neglect the issues during puberty and come for consultation when they are independent and employed. Most Indians come to a doctor when they are looking for alliances or during a relationship and are employed.

In any event, the causes of gynecomastia can be scientifically classified into two categories: primary and secondary.

Primary or idiopathic or physiological causes are the most common. It is seen in up to 90 percent of new-borns due to the transfer of hormones from the mother. New-born gynecomastia usually resolves spontaneously within four weeks of birth. Children with symptoms that persist after their first birthday should be examined further as they may be at risk of persistent pubertal gynecomastia. It is, however, important to rule out other causes when confronted with adolescent gynecomastia.

Secondary or non-physiological gynecomastia occurs due to a plethora of causes (etiologies) and requires thorough clinical and laboratory assessment (Table 1).

Table 1: Causes of Secondary Gynecomastia

1. Medication or drug abuse
Hormones: Androgens, anabolic steroids, oestrogens, oestrogenic agonists and hCG
Antiandrogens/Bicalutamide, flutamide, nilutamide, cyproterone and GRH agonists (leuprolide and goserelin)
Antibiotics: Metronidazole, ketoconazole, minocycline, isoniazid
Antiulcer medications: Cimetidine, ranitidine and omeprazole
Chemotherapeutic: Methotrexate, alkylating agents and vinca agents alkaloids

1. Medication or drug abuse

Cardiovascular drugs: Digoxin, ACEIs (Angiotensin-Converting Enzyme Inhibitors) (e.g., captopril and enalapril), calcium channel blockers (diltiazem, nifedipine, verapamil), amiodarone, methyldopa, spironolactone, reserpine and minoxidil

Psychoactive agents: Anxiolytic agents (e.g., diazepam), tricyclic antidepressants, phenothiazines, haloperidol and atypical antipsychotic agents

Miscellaneous: Antiretroviral therapy for HIV, metoclopramide, penicillamine, phenytoin, sulindac and Theophylline

2. Liver disorders like Cirrhosis

3. Hormonal issues:

3a. Primary hypogonadism

5α-reductase deficiency

Androgen insensitivity syndrome

Congenital anorchia

Hemochromatosis

Klinefelter syndrome

Testicular torsion

Testicular trauma

Viral orchitis

3b. Hormone producing Tumours

Adrenal tumours

Gastric carcinoma producing hCG

Large cell lung cancer-producing hCG

Pituitary tumours

Renal cell carcinoma producing hCG

Testicular tumours, particularly Leydig or Sertoli cell tumours

3c. Secondary hypogonadism

3d. Kallmann syndrome

4. Thyroid gland disorders like Hyperthyroidism

5. Kidney disorders like chronic renal insufficiency

6. Other rare causes
Familial gynecomastia
Malnutrition and disorders of impaired absorption (e.g., ulcerative colitis, cystic fibrosis)
Human immunodeficiency virus

Among the causes identified, one of the most prevalent is the use of **anabolic steroids**. The rate of occurrence of the various causes is related to the age of the population: use of anabolic steroids in younger patients and the use of pharmaceutical drugs and hypogonadism in older ones.

A study conducted in the Netherlands revealed that 96 percent of men who used steroids reported at least one side effect attributed to their use. Particularly common were acne, decreased libido, testicular atrophy and gynecomastia. A general distinction could be made between side effects that occur during a cycle of steroid therapyi.e. gynecomastia, fluid retention and aggressiveness—and those occurring after a cycle—i.e. erectile dysfunction and decreased libido.

A very systematic Canadian study about the effect of steroids on gynecomastia was published in the Annals of Plastic Surgery. It was observed that Anabolic-androgenic steroids (AAS) are widely implicated in gynecomastia development and surgery is the definitive treatment for cases persisting after cessation of AAS use.

In the study, a total of 964 cases were reviewed. Eleven percent (n = 105) of the patients had a history of AAS use. Compared with non-AAS users, AAS users were older at the time of gynecomastia onset (15 years versus 13 years; $P < 0.001$) and surgery (28 years versus 25 years; $P < 0.001$). The AAS users had a higher body mass index (27.3 kg/m2 versus 25.7 kg/m2; $P < 0.001$) and a greater proportion of patients self-identified as bodybuilders (40.0 percent versus 22.4 percent; P = 0.002). Although no difference was found in the excised bilateral mastectomy volume (92.1 cm3 versus 76.4 cm3; P = 0.20), the AAS users had significantly less lipoaspirate fat volume (250 mL versus 300 mL; P = 0.005). No difference was found in total complication rates. However, AAS users had significantly more revision mastectomy surgeries (3.8 percent versus 1.1 percent; P =0.02).

The conclusion of this study was that the unique breast composition of AAS users necessitates a surgical approach with meticulous intraoperative hemostasis and careful glandular removal to minimise recurrence and achieve comparable low complication rates.

Such cases of gynecomastia following drug use are increasing everywhere including in India. This is partly due to overzealous training for bodybuilding by self-proclaimed fitness specialists. However, the treatment remains **lipo-excision** like for any other scenario of gynecomastia.

While the definite cause of gynecomastia is rarely known, it is the surgeon's prerogative to assess and try ruling out secondary causes.

CLINICAL FEATURES AND ASSESSMENT

The clinical evaluation is mainly directed to rule out secondary causes and assess the severity of gynecomastia. It is important to review the patients' use of medications, supplements, and drug abuse. Symptoms that last longer than two years suggest unusual causes that require intervention for prompt resolution. Another major reason for intervention is the psychological effect of gynecomastia. The impact of gynecomastia is well-documented and warrants intervention along with counselling in many cases.

When the doctor examines a patient for the first time, he notes down various points from history like:

1. Duration of gynecomastia
2. History of any drugs or medicine that may lead to gynecomastia
3. Family history of gynecomastia
4. When was it first noticed and how it progressed
5. Whether it was painful or tender at any point
6. Any other clues to suggest other causes of gynecomastia
7. The patient's weight and history of major weight fluctuations
8. History of smoking, diabetes or any other factors that may affect the skin tone

When the doctor sees a patient with gynecomastia, the medical history is paramount as with any other medical condition. Many drugs may lead to gynecomastia as their side effect. These are primarily due to their effect on the various hormones in the blood. Most of these medications are the ones that have to been taken over long periods. Medicines cause gynecomastia through several mechanisms including the increase of serum oestrogen (feminine hormone) levels or oestrogen-like activity, decreased testosterone levels, hypogonadism (decreased function of male testes in terms of hormone production), anti-androgenic effects (reducing the effects of male hormones), etc. While the adverse effects of approved prescription and non-prescription drugs are fairly well-documented, little is known about the relationship between dietary supplements and gynecomastia. A recent study reported three cases of gynecomastia that appeared to have been caused by the application of products containing lavender oil and/or tea tree oil over the skin. Another product of concern is Androstenedione, also known as *Andro*. This is a commonly misused drug to enhance athletic performance and muscle bulk and endurance. It is converted to testosterone and is sold in health food stores as a natural substance designed to enhance athletic performance in males. This is not medically approved and is illegal. However, due to its effects on the feminine hormones, the males may experience feminisation and eventually gynecomastia. Many drugs used for treating high blood pressure, kidney disorders, fungal infection, epilepsy and heart issues have been implicated as a cause of gynecomastia.

One word of caution is that, just because the patient is on medication, it doesn't always mean that the breast has developed only due to the drug. Another way to assess is to possibly substitute the culprit medicine and watch for any reduction in the gland size. If it doesn't change in size even after discontinuation, then it is probably a coincidental finding and may not be the sole cause of gynecomastia. This method, however, is in no way fool-proof. Sometimes, laboratory tests are necessary for identifying the possible culprit.

Other than anabolic steroids, men who abuse alcohol, marijuana, heroin or amphetamines, should be alerted to the fact that gynecomastia could develop and take due note of any changes. Many recreational, addictive drugs act in the same way as the medical drugs in terms of their mode of causing gynecomastia—by causing fluctuations in hormone levels. There is a common misuse of the phrase, 'doobies make boobies'. While this statement inferring that all potheads gain feminine breasts is not entirely correct, Marijuana and other drugs are well-proven causes of gynecomastia. This is just another reason to stay away from pot.

Though there is a genetic component for gynecomastia, one cannot blame his dad for it. Except for some chromosomal anomalies and rare genetic mutations, gynecomastia is, for the most part, not genetic in inheritance.

Most men notice the gynecomastia lump during their high school years. It only later progresses in size. Initially, they do complain of pain and that's what brings the tissue to their attention. This is due to the florid nature (explained later) of the breast. But pain is an important symptom and should not be neglected. Breast lumps other than gynecomastia can present with a painful lump which we will discuss later.

Some men have what is called 'Runner's Nipple' or 'Jogger's Breast.' It is a condition where men who work out or jog a lot notice pain and tenderness (pain on touch) in the breast without any major abnormalities in the breast. Oddly enough, these people may even have a little blood oozing from the nipple. The condition called Mastodynia, which simply means 'breast pain,' is another rare presentation. The doctor will usually come to this rare diagnosis when all the tests have turned up negative and there is no attributable cause to the pain in the breast.

The local evaluation by the doctor should assess for nipple discharge, skin changes, breast masses, testicular masses and size. The physical examination should include evaluation of height and weight; and examination of the breasts, genitals, liver, body hair patterns, lymph nodes and thyroid. Assessment of symmetry and consistency of breast tissue is important. In a majority of cases, gynecomastia is on both sides (bilateral), although, sometimes, it can be present on only one side (unilateral). It is also important to rule out pseudo gynecomastia by assessing subareolar (under the nipple and areola) fat. Rarely, hard cancer masses along with the relevant skin changes may also be noted.

In our clinic, we note down points on an assessment sheet like this.

Table: 2 Pre-Surgical Gynecomastia Assessment Sheet

*Name: *Age:

*Weight: *Height:

*Secondary Sexual Characteristics: Normal/Abnormal

*Chest Circumference at Nipple level:

*Position of NAC in Relation to Mid-Arm Level:

*Grade of Gynecomastia:

*Status of Pectoralis Major: Normal/Hypotrophic/Hypertrophic

*Skin Pinch for Fat Assessment: Upper Chest Wall:

Lateral Chest Wall:

*Skin Tone: Right: Normal/Poor Left: Normal/Poor

*Direction of Skin Laxity: Both Inferior Quadrants/Both Inferior Quadrants with Lateral extension

*Accessory Chest Fat Folds: Present/Absent

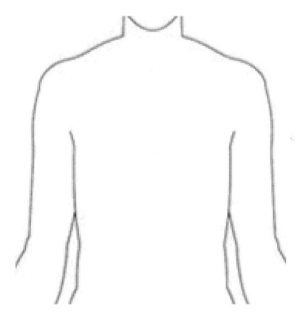

*Diagnosis: Idiopathic/Secondary Gynecomastia, Grade: I/ IIA/IIB/III

The findings and the extent of the gland are drawn on the outline diagram above.

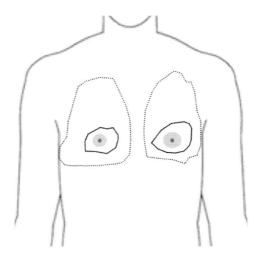

An example of pre-surgical marking. The difference in the sizes of areola
is noted and marked. The solid line is the extent of breast tissue and
the dotted line is the extent of the fat that needs to be even out during
liposuction. Note the asymmetries in the extent of gland and fat

In most cases, gynecomastia is a purely cosmetic issue and the targets
of correction are:

1. Achieve a better overall shape of the chest.

2. Achieve symmetry between either side.

3. Minimise the risk of complications.

As it is primarily a cosmetic issue, the treating doctor does have to
note many factors to devise a meticulous and detailed surgical plan.

Among the basic measurements are the weight and height of the
patient. Weight and the history of weight fluctuations give us an insight
into the fitness levels and lifestyle of the patient. Sometimes, they may
even point to an underlying endocrine/hormonal issue especially in
men with subtle thyroid hormonal disorders. If someone has lost a lot
of weight in the recent past, expect to see a lot of stretch marks and a
considerable amount of loose skin. The contrary is true too. In men
who have worked out a lot, one may notice stretch marks along the side
of the chest extending to the shoulders. It is important to note that they
are often unrelated to gynecomastia and may not reduce after surgery.

As gynecomastia can occur due to hormonal disturbances, the doctor does look for any clinical signs pointing to them. Also, it is important to determine the sexual maturity of the individual. Sexual maturity is classified into five stages depending on genital and pubic hair development. This assessment by visual inspection was described by Marshall and Tanner.

The stages of genital maturity were graded separately from pubic hair growth as follows

Stage 1: The testes, scrotum and penis are about the same size and proportion as in early childhood

Stage 2: The scrotum and testes enlarge and the scrotal sac reddens and changes in texture. There is little to no enlargement of the penis.

Stage 3: There is further growth of the testes and scrotum and the penis begins to enlarge, mainly in length.

Stage 4: The testes and scrotum continue to enlarge and the scrotal skin continues to darken. The penis continues to grow in breadth and length with the development of the glans.

Stage 5: The genitalia are of adult size and shape. No further enlargement takes place.

Pubic hair was staged as follows:

Stage 1: The vellus (tiny uncoloured hair) of the pubis resembles that over the abdomen.

Stage 2: Sparse growth of long, slightly pigmented, downy hair, straight or only slightly curled, appears chiefly at the base of the penis.

Stage 3: The hair is considerably darker, courser and more curled. It spreads sparsely over the junction of the pubis.

Stage 4: The hair is now adult-like but the area covered is still considerably smaller than in most adults. There is no spread to the medial surface of the thighs.

Stage 5: The hair is adult in quantity and type, distributed in the "male" pattern of an inverse triangle and may spread to the medial surface of the thighs.

These stages are again important to assess for the signs the hormonal issues and sexual maturity which may be inter-related. These clinical signs form what is commonly called the secondary sexual characteristics. The sexual characteristics are controlled by hormones which distinguish between sexually mature males and females but are not directly involved in reproduction are hence called secondary sexual characteristics. The doctor would also look for body hair pattern like on the chest, facial hair (beard), frontal balding on the scalp, prominence of Adam's apple, the pitch of the voice (low pitched deeper voice in mature males), etc. All these do provide clues to any hormonal issues and, if found, may need further hormonal assessment via blood tests which in turn may require an endocrinologist's consultation.

Though gynecomastia is usually on both sides, its is very rarely symmetric. Most of the patients have gross or at least minimal visible differences between either sides. It is very important the doctor notices them and points them out to the patient too. Sometimes, the differences are so subtle that the patient himself may not have noticed them. The difference between the right and left may be in terms of the amount of breast tissues, its location in relation to the nipple, its extent towards to the side of the chest, position of the nipple and areolae, projection of both the sides when viewed from the side, size of muscles of either side, etc.

The nipple and areola may also be asymmetric. The ideal position of the nipple is at the mid-arm level. The mid-arm level is the point between the topmost part of the shoulder and the elbow. When you draw a line across the point onto the chest, you will mark the ideal nipple position. But there is a wide variation in the nipple position among men and many a time the abnormal position goes unnoticed.

Even in men with perfectly symmetric breast tissue, the nipple and the areola may be asymmetric. I have noticed men having differences in either side like a more projecting nipple on one side, larger areola on one side, difference in the colour of areola, a subtle folding in the areolar skin, a higher placed nipple on one side, a nipple located more on the side and so many other subtle differences. It is important to note that not all of them can be corrected by the gynecomastia surgery alone. Most differences are so subtle that many men don't mind it before or after the procedure. Note the asymmetry in gynecomastia in the pictures below:

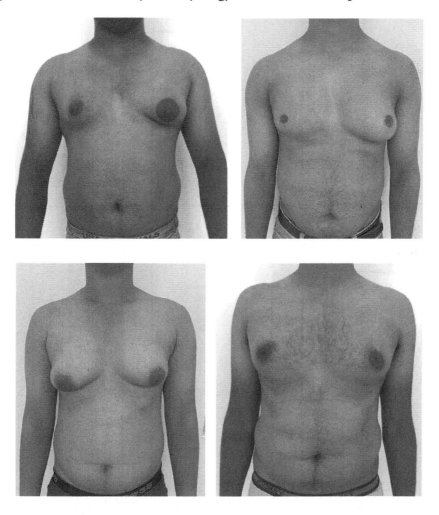

Note the asymmetry between the two sides in terms of the breast tissue, areola and nipple

Another variable before assessing the symmetry or the lack of it is to assess the position of the shoulders. Many right-handed people will have a slightly lower right shoulder as compared to the left. Also, most right-handed people have a slightly bigger right-side chest muscle (pectoralis major muscle). It's important to factor in these normal but important differences between both the sides before devising a surgical plan.

It is also important to notice the amount of overall fat and the fat distribution patterns in the patient. Many people have asymmetric fat deposition and fat folds too. The amount of fat gives us an idea about the overall fat distribution patterns, fitness level of the patient and the amount of fat that needs to be removed during the procedure for a better result. The fat is assessed by what's called the skin pick test wherein the skin, along with the fat below it, is pinched to get an idea of the thickness of the fat fold in a particular area. A more objective way is to use calipers and measure the fat.

Skin tone is an assessment that's mandatory but is often overlooked. When you pinch your skin on any part of the body, the skin snaps back into place almost instantly. The speed at which it snaps back gives us a clue into the tone of the skin in that particular area. The skin tone is due to the microstructure of the dermis (the inner white part of skin under the outer visible layer) and the amount of collagen in it. Following loss of a lot of weight, or after pregnancy, the appearance of stretch marks indicates a reduction of skin tone in that area. The skin tone is also important in determining how well the skin will shrink and reshape itself when the breast tissue is removed. The skin tone is also determined by the amount of breast tissue underneath. Sometimes, the breast tissue is so much that it has stretched the overlying skin enough to reduce its tone to a large extent. This may again compromise skin retraction/reshaping after surgery. Smokers, diabetics and people who use steroids for any reason have generally poorer skin tone. As the grade of gynecomastia increases, the chances of loose skin and subsequently reduced skin tone also increases. The skin issues sometimes have to be dealt with in separate surgeries or non-surgical procedures depending on the amount of laxity in the skin. To take skin tone into factoring when grading gynecomastia, I had to revise the existing gynecomastia grading. It was published in the Brazilian Journal of plastic surgery. You will read more about it later on.

Also, equally paramount is to note the direction of skin laxity. Many men have loose skin over the lower part of the breast that extends to the side of the chest. Others may have looseness all over especially in grade III gynecomastia. The direction is again important in planning the future surgery in terms of the surgical scars that may be left behind. Associated with these loose skin folds are folds of fat. Many men have two or even three fat folds on the side of the chest that make the treatment a little more elaborate and need more assessment. But most men have a single fold extending from the lower breast to the side of the chest. Men who are fit or skinny have no folds at all and are the simplest to manage.

Also, note is made of evidence of liver disease or kidney disorders— for example, palmar erythema (excess redness of palms), bruising, spider nevi (visible abnormal veins), liver enlargement, etc.

Evidence to suggest inadequate levels of testosterone is hairless, shiny skin; decreased testicular size; testicular masses; and a feminine voice. The presence of varicocele has also been strongly associated with gynecomastia.

Chapter 2

GRADING AND TYPES OF GYNECOMASTIA

If there is one factor that determines the kind of surgery that needs to be done and also determines the outcomes; it the grade of gynecomastia. Though there are many different methods of grading gynecomastia, the most commonly followed is Simon's grading described in 1973. He classified gynecomastia into three grades depending on the amount of breast tissue and loose skin on top of the breast.

- Grade I: Small enlargement without skin excess
- Grade IIa: Moderate enlargement without skin excess
- Grade IIb: Moderate enlargement with minor skin excess
- Grade III: Marked enlargement with a lot of excess skin, resembling a female breast

Observe the pictures of various grades below.

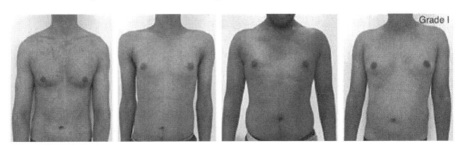

Grade I Gynecomastia

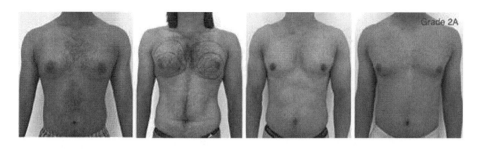

Grade IIA Gynecomastia

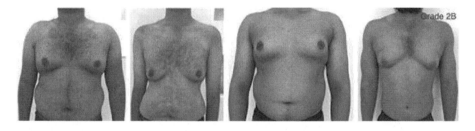

Grade IIB Gynecomastia

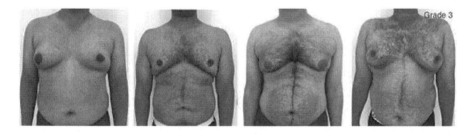

Grade III Gynecomastia

Rohrich in 2003 proposed another classification into four grades.

- Grade I: Minimal hypertrophy (< 250 g) without ptosis
- Grade II: Moderate hypertrophy (250–500 g) without ptosis
- Grade III: Severe hypertrophy (> 500 g) with grade I ptosis
- Grade IV: Severe hypertrophy with grade II or grade III ptosis

Though these two are used worldwide, Simon's grading is simple and used more widely. One addition I would like to suggest to these gradings is the addition of skin tone factor. To put it simply, while skin excess is the loose skin on top of the breast tissue, skin tone is the inherent capacity of the skin to shrink and contract after the surgery. While skin excess has a linear progression from grades 1 to 3, skin tone can be independent of it.

The revised grading could be something like this:

- Grade IT: Small enlargement, no skin excess, normal skin tone

- Grade 1L: Small enlargement, no skin excess, poor skin tone

- Grade IIAT: Moderate enlargement, no skin excess, normal skin tone

- Grade IIAL: Moderate enlargement, no skin excess, poor skin tone

- Grade IIBT: Moderate enlargement, minimal skin excess, normal skin tone

- Grade IIBL: Moderate enlargement, minimal skin excess, poor skin tone

- Grade IIIT: Marked enlargement, lot of excess skin, normal skin tone

- Grade IIIL: Marked enlargement, lot of excess skin, poor skin tone

The 'L' here would indicate laxity, meaning poor skin tone. This revised grading would also predict the eventual surgical results in terms of skin reshaping more accurately. And, once documented into history, it would serve as a reminder about the patient's original skin tone before the surgery and during follow-up. This revised grading was published by the author in the Brazilian Journal of plastic surgery in 2019.

This is very important and is very often understated for reasons I cannot fathom. When two patients with grade IIA come for surgery and get operated by the same technique under the same surgeon, the results may be different—the reason being the difference in skin tone between the two. This should not come as a surprise as such a difference in results follows other surgeries like liposuction too. The lack of skin tone makes a visible difference in the results after any procedure. A patient with loose skin after surgery who seemingly had normal skin may need other non-non-surgical procedures or, very rarely, surgery to tighten the loose skin. This can happen even in Grade IIA Gynecomastia. This can happen when the skin tone is not assessed.

Commonly, three clinical types of gynecomastia have been described. The type is usually related to the duration of the appearance of the breast and its pattern when one examines under a microscope.

1. Florid type: It is characterised by an increase in ductal tissue (breast tissue) and vascularity, meaning it has more blood supply than usual. A variable amount of fat tends to be mixed in with the ductal tissue, which is usually seen when the duration is four months or less. It is usually the first to appear. Sometimes, this type can be painful and tender to touch. However, the pain and tenderness reduce with time even without any treatment.

2. Fibrous type: It has more stromal fibrosis and a few ducts, usually present after one year. It is much harder to feel and not usually painful. It has harder tissue and feels like thick firm tissue resembling the tip of the nose sometimes.

3. Intermediate type: It is a mixture of these two. The intermediate type is thought to be a progression from florid to fibrous and is usually seen between four and 12 months of the appearance of gynecomastia.

Though normally X-rays, mammograms or ultrasound are not advised for gynecomastia, the pattern on such tests does reveal some interesting facts about the structure of gynecomastia. Three radiological patterns of gynecomastia have been normally described:

1. Nodular pattern: It is seen in the early florid phase. The mammogram shows a disc-shaped, evenly dense, well-circumscribed opacity that may have some irregularities. The ultrasound demonstrates a hypoechoic (which means that the tissue is less dense) mass beneath the nipple surrounded by fatty tissue.

2. Dendritic pattern: When this is seen, it means that the breast is in an irreversible, chronic, fibrotic phase. The mammogram shows an irregular wedge-shaped lump with its apex behind the areola and then extensions radiating into the deep fat tissue, mainly in the upper outer parts of the chest.

3. Diffuse glandular pattern: This consists of an overall increase in breast size that presents identically on mammography and sonography to the female dense heterogeneous breast. This means it looks like an exact female breast on the scans.

Though these patterns may seem redundant and futile to the patient, it does reveal a tight correlation between how a gland develops, how it presents clinically and how it looks on the scans. It also tells us that what you diagnose clinically most often is reflected on the scans too. That is one of the reasons scans are not generally advised when we clinically diagnose gynecomastia. Scans, however, become important when one comes across unusual findings like:

1. Unusually hard breast tissue

2. Breast tissue that feels different in different areas

3. Unnaturally immobile tissue. Means it is fixed to the underlying muscle or the skin overlying it

4. Nipple discharge of any kind or ulcers

5. Enlarged lymph nodes in the armpits

6. A breast that pulls the skin towards it, meaning the tissue is abnormally active

The doctor would look for these signs and advise scans to rule out cancers. These are very rare but should nevertheless be looked out for. These become even more important in people with risk factors for breast cancer like old age; genetic factors like Klinefelter syndrome or rare mutations; history of chest radiation; occupational exposure to heat or exhaust gas; patients taking oestrogen; testicular disease like Crypotorchidism; history of removal of testes; inguinal hernia by birth; injury to testes; liver diseases; obesity, etc. We will discuss more about male breast cancer later on.

Chapter 3

DIAGNOSIS AND WORK-UP

Though the clinical diagnosis of gynecomastia is straightforward, some issues may make this seemingly simple issue a little tricky. Such diagnoses that closely mimic a certain other disorder are called differential diagnoses.

One such common differential diagnosis is pseudo gynecomastia. As the name suggests, it refers to 'false male breast,' meaning fat that masquerades as breast tissue. It is especially common in men who are overweight or obese. However, in my opinion, the term pseudo gynecomastia is overused and over-diagnosed. There have been instances in mine and my colleagues' practices where a patient is referred to us as pseudo gynecomastia and the patient is expecting liposuction as the sole treatment.

Some surgeons have even gone ahead and done liposuction to this pseudo gynecomastia only to then realise that there is a large amount of breast tissue left. Now, this complicates the issue manifold. One, the patient has not been told that he requires a gland excision and a bigger skin cut to do the same. Now, either the surgeon has to explain to the patient's friends or relatives that the surgical plan has changed as he has now noticed breast tissue or he has to end the procedure there and plan breast tissue removal later on. In either of these scenarios, the surgeon does not come off with flying colours. More importantly, the patient is put through a procedure that he is ill-prepared for.

If the surgeon takes the relatives into confidence and goes ahead and operates, removing the breast tissue, it is left to him to explain it to the patient when he comes out of anaesthesia. The matter is easier said than done as it depends entirely on how the patient takes the news. If the surgeon chooses the second option and ends the surgery without removing the gland, he needs to explain that to the patient who may not be happy on hearing that he needs another procedure to sort out his chest. I have seen patients who underwent only liposuction for 'pseudo gynecomastia' and came to me complaining that their surgeon has left a lot of hard fat under the nipple. I have had to explain to such patients that only fat was removed and the breast tissue was left behind and, indeed, the diagnosis may be wrong. Now imagine the patient's conundrum at this phase. An issue that could have been easily sorted in the first procedure has now dragged on, not only needing another procedure but also making the patient invest a disproportionate amount of time to sort out the one issue at hand.

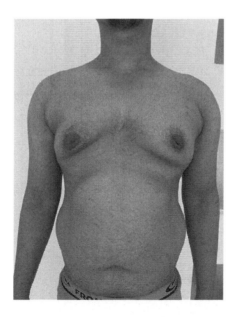

An example of someone diagnosed as pseudo gynecomastia, was planned for liposuction and, intra-operatively, the decision was changed to remove the gland. Note the persistent gland and loose skin. Such cases would be easily avoided by a proper diagnosis and treatment plan.

This is especially true if the patient, following liposuction, gets fitter and loses more weight only to notice his breast tissue getting more prominent. Before the surgery and his weight loss, the overall smooth contour due to fat might have camouflaged the breast tissue better than when he gets the liposuction or loses weight. All these issues are readily avoided if one is careful in diagnosing pseudo gynecomastia. If the diagnosis is correct, then liposuction should suffice.

This diagnosis is especially important as pseudo gynecomastia does not require surgery in many cases as diet and exercise my dissolve the fat. Gynecomastia, however, requires surgery to treat it and exercise or diet will never suffice.

Apart from fat, there may be other swellings on the chest that simulate gynecomastia. These swellings may arise from any of the structures over the chest. In most cases, they are unilateral, meaning they are usually only on one side. Nonetheless, it is paramount to diagnoses the swelling before proceeding with the treatment plan.

Skin swellings are quite common on the chest too. The most common among them is the lipoma. It is an accumulation of immature, abnormal fat cells under the skin. They are more mobile under the skin than the breast tissue and are softer. The treatment for these lipomas is excision (removal) through a small cut in the skin. A big enough lipoma can mimic a breast. Many other such swellings can occur on the chest skin, like a sebaceous cyst, dermoid cysts, fat necrosis after injury (where the fat cells die in a particular area following a high impact injury and clump up), etc. Most of them are quite straightforward for the doctor to rule them out.

Another sometimes serious and under-diagnosed issue is mastitis. It is an infection of the breast tissue. It is way more common in females but does occasionally affect men with breasts. The breast glands can get infected by various paths. It can get infected through external sources across the skin, like an injury to the skin, nipple piercings or just a skin infection that spreads inwards. The other mode is infection via blood. Any infection in a part of the body can theoretically spread to another tissue like the breast. When one has mastitis they would complain of severe pain, redness over the chest skin, occasional pus discharge from the nipple, enlarged lymph nodes in the armpits (axilla) and fever. The treatment is a course of antibiotics and occasionally removal of the pus and if necessary, the gland.

The word 'tumour' incites various unpleasant feelings in people. They vary from shock to distress. But not all tumours are cancers and not all cancers are untreatable. Most tumours are benign, meaning, non-cancerous. They are treated like any other swelling and usually require removal. I have patients coming in for consultation with a family history of cancer; they are unusually worked up about gynecomastia. Such patients need to be reassured but evaluated nonetheless. In the breast tissue, some men do develop breast cysts and fibroadenomas.

Breast cysts are fluid-filled swellings that have a thin capsule. These cysts again are commoner in females and show up as lumps on examination. In most cases, an ultrasound is required to correctly diagnose the issue. Sometimes, your doctor will insert a thin needle into the breast lump and attempt to withdraw (aspirate) the fluid. This may be done under ultrasound guidance or by feeling the lump itself. If the fluid comes out and the breast lump goes away, your doctor can make a diagnosis of the breast cyst immediately. If the fluid is not bloody and the breast lump disappears, you need no further testing or treatment unless it comes back. If the fluid appears bloody or the breast lump doesn't disappear, your doctor may send a sample of the fluid for lab testing and refer you to a radiologist for the scans. If no fluid is withdrawn, your doctor will likely recommend a scan such as a diagnostic mammogram and or ultrasound. Lack of fluid or a breast lump that doesn't disappear after aspiration suggests that the breast lump, or at least a portion of it, is solid and a sample of these cells may be collected to check for cancer (fine-needle aspiration biopsy). The treatment of breast cysts is rarely by surgery. It is operated upon only if the diagnosis is unclear even with the scans or if it is troublesome to the patient.

Other breast swellings that may occur in a male breast are duct ectasia, fibroadenoma and breast cancers. While duct ectasia and fibroadenomas are benign, cancer is another matter altogether. Men with duct ectasia may have bloody nipple discharge that many find scary. One fine day, the individual wakes up to find a bloodstain on his nipple. Many men freak out and rush to the doctor fearing cancer. It usually is a duct ectasia which is nothing but alteration in the ductal structure in the breast. It sometimes needs treatment but always needs assessment. Cancer should always be ruled out when there is a nipple discharge.

Fibroadenomas are the most common swellings in a female breast. Some do occur in men. They feel like a firm lump that is unnaturally mobile. It was often referred to as the 'mouse in the breast.' While that scenario is far-fetched for a male breast, nonetheless, it depicts how mobile a fibroadenoma can be. The treatment is removal if the size is more than three centimetres in diameter. Occasionally, men do wait for them to get very big, assuming it's just a skin lump. While it's not necessarily dangerous, it's always better to know what it is than just wait unknowingly.

Gretchen Dickson, in 2012, published a widely referenced article in the journal 'American Family Physician' that outlined an algorithm to diagnose gynecomastia.

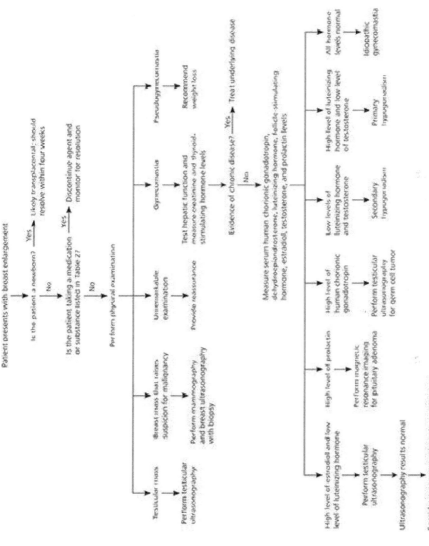

When one talks about tests for a gynecomastia patient, it has two facets to it

1. Tests to check for causes of gynecomastia
2. Test mandatory to check if the patient is fit for surgery

Once the doctor suspects gynecomastia, then the next step is to check if there is indeed a hormonal issue or it is idiopathic. The word idiopathic itself means that the cause is unknown. It accounts for over 70 to 90 percent of all cases of gynecomastia. However, before diagnosing someone as 'Idiopathic Gynecomastia' the doctor needs to rule out a few things. 'Secondary Gynecomastia' is when there is a proven cause for gynecomastia as was enlisted above.

Apart from the drug-induced gynecomastia that may be easier to diagnoses, the doctor should bear in mind other hormonal disorders. Laboratory evaluation is indicated only if the clinical assessment suggests a secondary underlying cause. It is not needed for boys at puberty for enlargement due to fat (pseudo gynecomastia) and for men taking drugs known to cause gynecomastia.

In cases of secondary gynecomastia, without a clear cause, laboratory tests should be advised and must include, liver, kidney and thyroid function tests (to exclude the respective causative medical conditions), as well as hormonal tests. The hormonal analysis, if necessary, is always a group of tests. They include:

1. Oestrogen level
2. Total and free testosterone
3. Luteinising hormone
4. Follicle stimulating hormone
5. Prolactin
6. And occasionally hCG, DHEASO4 or 17 ketosteroids, SHBG and αFetoprotein

7. If the patient's testes are small, the patient's karyotype (chromosomal analysis) should be done to exclude Klinefelter's Syndrome.

If all tests are negative, the patient should be diagnosed with Idiopathic Gynecomastia. Sometimes, it is indeed advisable to have an endocrinologist look at such patients as there may be other important issues than just gynecomastia. It is especially more prudent to meet one if these tests reveal significant variations. Early stages of secondary gynecomastia can be medically treated though the gland does not always regress and may end up needing a procedure eventually to sort out the gland.

Ultrasonography and mammography can occasionally be used to differentiate fat from breast tissue or if there are abnormal masses especially in terms of consistency. Scans are needed when the patient has one of the signs suggestive of a cancer lump. Other than these, scans may be necessary to ascertain if the breast tissue feels abnormal or irregular in places. Mammography is about 90 percent sensitive and 90 percent specific for cancers compared to benign masses in men.

However, biopsy is the only way to make a definitive diagnosis. Patients with a hard, irregular or asymmetrical mass; nipple discharge (bloody or non-bloody); enlarged armpit lymph nodes; or a mass fixed to skin or the chest wall must have a biopsy. Usually, a core biopsy is recommended over the fine-needle or excisional biopsy. In core biopsy, a small amount of tissue is taken via a small hole under local anaesthesia. It is more accurate over the commonly done fine-needle biopsy. In a fine-needle biopsy, an injection is given and the cells obtained through it are examined under a microscope. Since the amount of cells one gets from such biopsy is very small, the chances of error are consequently high. An excision biopsy is one where the lump is removed in its entirety and sent for testing. While this is the most accurate, it is reserved for specific cases where the diagnosis with routine biopsies is not confirmatory.

Rarely done tests include:

Ultrasound of testes: If there is any abnormality in the testes on examination or if there is a raised beta-hCG or alpha-fetoprotein.

Abdominal Scans: If a tumour of the adrenal glands or the testes is thought to be responsible for the gynecomastia after hormonal analysis.

Chest X-ray: If a lung tumour is suspected as a cause for gynecomastia. Sometimes, tumours in other tissues may be hormonally active, meaning they may produce hormones which in turn may lead to gynecomastia. Though these are rare, one does come across such cases and is quite often a diagnostic dilemma.

Once these diagnostic tests are done as necessary, the next set of tests is for those planning to undergo the corrective procedures. Since the procedures can be theoretically done under local or general anaesthesia, the tests also vary depending on the anaesthesia planned. For a gynecomastia surgery under local anaesthesia, no additional tests are normally needed if the patient is clinically fit and has a clear unremarkable history. When the procedure is planned under general anaesthesia, a set of tests is mandatory.

1. Complete blood counts.

2. Blood sugar levels.

3. Coagulation parameters: PT, INR, and aPTT.

4. Kidney function tests: Serum Creatinine and Urea levels.

5. Other tests that are often done are: HIV screening, HBsAg to check for hepatitis B, HCV, etc.

6. Apart from these routine tests, a few more may be advised depending on the patient's age, medical history, and the factors.

These include Echocardiography, Chest X-rays, ECG, Liver function tests, Sickle cell tests, etc. Cardiac (heart) evaluation becomes necessary when an older patient comes for corrective surgery. Occasionally a consultation with a cardiologist or the relevant physician is needed before surgery.

Chapter 4
TREATMENT

Patients with gynecomastia explore treatments most commonly for cosmetic reasons. The reason they get it done is to look better and achieve a positive outlook once done. Pain is more common in patients with gynecomastia that is rapidly progressive or of recent onset and is very rarely the precursor for surgery. For patients with secondary gynecomastia, treatment is aimed at improving the underlying illness or discontinuing the use of the culprit medication. Watchful waiting with regular follow-up is appropriate for those with Physiologic gynecomastia who are untroubled by symptoms and who have no features that suggest underlying disease or malignancy. The wait-and-watch policy is needed when someone even with a large breast is untroubled by it psychologically. Sometimes, even breasts that are not all that big during puberty may need to be operated upon. This scenario is a recurring one where a teenager comes across as mildly depressed due to his gynecomastia though, clinically, it may just be grade one. There is, however, a strong correlation between the size of one's gynecomastia and how much it affects them. There is definite merit in operating on such patients to better their psychological outlook if for nothing else.

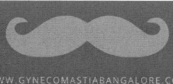

WWW.GYNECOMASTIABANGALORE.COM

BENEFITS OF GYNECOMASTIA SURGERY

 GET A MASCULINE PHYSIQUE

 VISIBLE RESULTS OF PECTORAL MUSCLE SHAPE

 MOTIVATION TO MAINTAIN A HEALTHY BODY WEIGHT & LIFESTYLE

 AUGMENTED SELF-ESTEEM

 IMPROVED CONFIDENCE WEARING SWIMSUITS OR DURING INTIMACY

 BETTER ABILITY TO WEAR FITTED SHIRTS

 BETTER COMFORT IN DAY-TO-DAY LIFE

Join the conversation!

Contact us at +91 7022543542

- Better comfort in day-to-day life.
- Better ability to wear fitted shirts.
- Improved confidence wearing swimsuits or during intimacy.
- Augmented self-esteem.
- Motivation to maintain a healthy body weight & lifestyle.
- Visible results of pectoral muscle shape.
- Get a masculine physique.

Medications are more effective if used as early as possible after symptoms are first noticed, whereas surgery can be performed at any time with similar results. The more delayed the gynecomastia consultation, the bigger it is in size, the firmer the gland is, the lesser chances of it improving any significantly with medications.

New-onset gynecomastia (<6 months of duration) often reduces in teenagers and, many a time, only a follow-up is necessary. This protocol is more accurate if the gland is small, like in grade one. Even in some adults who are not unduly bothered by it, live all their life with the breast and wouldn't mind having them. In such cases, of course, reassurance is sufficient except in cases with cosmetic concerns. However, if gynecomastia persists for more than one year, instances of complete reduction are very less and close to nil. This persistence is due to the predominance of dense fibrous tissue which is never going to reduce on its own. If gynecomastia persists and is associated with severe pain, tenderness and psychological distress, treatment is necessary.

Treatment also depends on the cause and the extent to which the individual is affected. If gynecomastia is drug-induced, symptoms may regress when the appropriate medication is stopped or changed. Gynecomastia secondary of systemic illnesses often regresses with the treatment of these disorders. For example, the treatment of hyperthyroidism—or the surgical removal of testicular, adrenal or other causative tumours—may lead to spontaneous reduction.

MEDICAL TREATMENT

In a nutshell, no medical treatment causes complete regression of gynecomastia. It may only provide partial regression or symptomatic relief and, that too, in selected patients. The medical treatment options focus on reversing the effect of hormonal changes on the breast. These options are androgens, antioestrogens and aromatase inhibitors. These drugs are to be used only with a prescription and in carefully selected individuals. They come with their side effects if used unwisely.

Once we do come across a suitable patient and where we see that there is a high possibility that the gynecomastia may spontaneously regress, the decision on when to treat is also often tricky and challenging. However, medical treatment is likely to be beneficial if implemented during the early proliferative phase, before the glandular structure is gradually replaced by stromal hyalinisation and fibrosis (meaning, the gland has not hardened yet). Androgens, antioestrogens and aromatase inhibitors have been tested for gynecomastia treatment with varying success in different scenarios.

1. Danazol: It is a synthetic steroid-like drug with an anti-gonadotropic effect. It reduces the activity of gonadotrophin hormones—Follicle stimulating hormone (FSH) and Luteinising Hormone (LH). It reduces the stimulatory effects of oestrogens over the breast tissue. A daily dose of 200 to 600 milligrams has been tried in many studies. While it has proven beneficial to an extent, there was a high relapse rate. What it means is that, once you stop the drug, the breast tissue tends to grow back to its initial size. Though the side effects are not too

troublesome, the high chances of relapse make it an unattractive treatment option.

2. Tamoxifen: It is an antioestrogen drug. It again reduces the effect of feminine hormones on the body. It is commonly used for breast cancer treatment in females and can also occasionally be used as an alternative to surgery to treat gynecomastia. It is used in doses of 10 to 40 milligrams per day in adolescent males under the age of 20 for one to 12 months. The reduction in breast pain is noted in around 80 percent of the cases and approximately 80 percent see a decrease in the swelling. The response is dependent on the duration of the treatment. Moreover, the chances of re-occurrence of glands also depend on the length of therapy. It also appears to be most effective within the first six months of gynecomastia when the breast tissue growth is most abundant and before fibrosis occurs. Furthermore, in two studies involving patients who developed gynecomastia, following treatment for prostatic cancer, Tamoxifen was shown to be an effective treatment. Based on the data above and the overall safety of the drug, it is not unreasonable to try a three-month course of Tamoxifen therapy in selected patients with painful gynecomastia of recent onset.

It belongs to a group of drugs called Selective Oestrogen Receptor Modulators (SERM) of which Raloxifene is another. It, too, has shown similar effects on the breast tissue. Breast tissue reduced spontaneously in up to half of the cases. Recurrence of gynecomastia may occur in up to 25 percent of the cases after Tamoxifen is stopped. So, a further course for six months is indicated for non-responders. But these drugs should be used very judiciously and we do need more trials to once and for all prove its role in gynecomastia management. Two studies have compared Tamoxifen with other medical therapies. In conclusion, while Tamoxifen is more beneficial than Danazol and Raloxifene is better than Tamoxifen, they are still unproven in the long-term and large, multicentre trials. To date, no medical agents for treating gynecomastia have been approved in the United States by the Food and Drug Administration (FDA). Given the small sample sizes and inadequacy of the methodology of current research, there is no consensus regarding either the drug of choice or the optimal duration of treatment.

3. Clomiphene citrate: It is used for its antioestrogen effects and has been tested as a treatment of pubertal gynecomastia in a total of three studies with variable results. Increasing the dose of clomiphene to 100 milligrams per day for a total of six months was associated with complete resolution of signs in 64 percent of patients. There were no significant side effects, although nausea, rashes and visual problems were noticed with this drug in other settings. However, the chances of re-occurrence of the gland are poorly documented in long-term studies.

4. Testosterone: It was one of the first drugs tried in treating gynecomastia. In patients with hypogonadism, testosterone replacement usually improves gynecomastia, but there is no data for the use of androgens in males with a typical hormonal profile. In these patients, testosterone replacement may worsen the gynecomastia because of the aromatisation (conversion) of testosterone to oestrogen. When you take testosterone, and if your blood testosterone levels are already normal, the excess gets converted to female hormones and will, in fact, worsen gynecomastia. So, don't go and buy these injections that seem to circulate in the black market, especially around gyms.

5. Aromatase Inhibitors: These drugs block oestrogen synthesis and decrease the oestrogen to androgen ratio. Anastrozole is the one usually used and is a potent, highly selective aromatase inhibitor that decreases the oestrogen concentration in males. Testolactone is an aromatase inhibitor tested in a small, uncontrolled trial of pubertal gynecomastia. The use of aromatase inhibitors is supported by incomplete evidence and hence the potential benefits against the side effects should be considered before starting treatment. Aromatase inhibitors are widely prescribed for hormone-responsive breast cancers in older, postmenopausal women. It is well-known that aromatase inhibition results in a dramatic reduction of tumour oestrogen concentrations and has a specific role there, but its role in gynecomastia is far from clear. Anastrozole was also studied in a group of prostate cancer patients treated with bicalutamide, a drug that causes gynecomastia. A dose of one milligram daily appeared to be mildly effective against the appearance of gynecomastia. Tamoxifen was much more effective, however, in the prevention of gynecomastia in these men. Due to these disappointing results, aromatase inhibitors are not recommended as a first-line treatment for any gynecomastia in men.

SURGERY

"He has breasts. Just take them out, doc," said a patient's father to me during his 22-year-old son's consultation. That was his first sentence, even before I had explained to him anything about the procedure or even diagnosis. Well, as I explained to them later on, there is more to it than just 'taking it out'.

The first surgical treatment of gynecomastia is credited to Paulas Aegineta (625–690 AD), a Byzantine Greek physician who performed the surgery through a cut below the breast. Webster in

1946, described semicircular intra-areolar incision. Current surgical techniques favour standard liposuction/suction-assisted lipectomy (SAL) and ultrasound-assisted liposuction (UAL) with a combination of removal of breast tissue with the advantage of tackling both the fat in the chest along with the breast tissue.

Before one sets out to correct the gynecomastia, the goals should be borne in mind:

1. Achieve a better chest shape.

2. Achieve symmetry as much as possible between either side.

3. Correct the loose skin in one or two stages depending on the grade of gynecomastia.

4. Correct the position of the nipple and areola complex (NAC).

5. Minimise scarring.

6. Minimise post-procedure complications and achieve a speedy recovery.

Surgery should be considered in patients with cosmetic concern, discomfort, psychological stress, long-standing gynecomastia (>12m) and suspected cancers. In general, all grades of gynecomastia are treated with a combination of liposuction and excision (removal of the gland), called lipo-excision. This combination is right, even for grades I and II. In patients with Simon grade III, any form of liposuction is usually combined with skin resection but, sometimes, these are also done separately after the lipo-excision. The skin resection may be delayed in most cases to wait for skin retraction and subsequently reduce the amount of surgical scarring. In these severe cases, several types of incisions have been reported. For example, circum-areolar incision encompassing the superior or inferior half of the areola, omega incision, concentric circles incision and inframammary incision. In some cases, the nipple-areolar complex is transferred on its blood supply or rarely repositioned as a full-thickness skin graft. We shall be discussing all these aspects in detail as we go on.

The minimum age at which the surgery can be done is hotly debated. The general consensus is that, if the gynecomastia is significant and affects the psychology of the individual, then it can be done in early teens too. Gynecomastia is a cause of considerable psycho-social discomfort, stress and worsening of self-image in adolescent boys. It is essential to understand these concerns to provide proper management. Many parents casually neglect the issues raised by the boys only later to realise the psychological effects of a poor body image.

Once you do decide on getting the gynecomastia surgery done, you must research the prospective surgeons. Here are a few steps-by-step pointers to finding your gynecomastia surgeon.

1. Perform a Google search of the gynecomastia surgeons in your area. A word-of-mouth reference is better.

2. Check the surgeon's gynecomastia surgery website gallery, which would have 'before and after' pictures, and assess the results yourself.

3. Shortlist the surgeons who you feel are experts.

4. Check their Board Certification Degrees.

5. Look for MCh or DNB degrees that are valid in Indian Boards.

6. Make a list of questions that you will ask your surgeon.

7. Meet a few surgeons who you think fit the above criteria.

8. Take your time during the consultation and clarify all your doubts.

9. Check how frankly the surgeon discusses his experience and complications.

10. Check if his surgical technique is the latest.

11. Check if the surgeon has international experience and scientific publications.

12. The often-underestimated subjective factor is just how comfortable you felt with your surgeon.

Many parents attribute adolescent gynecomastia to fat. A rapid increase in obesity among children and adolescents results in a higher number of patients presenting with breast enlargement and disproportionate diagnoses of 'pseudo gynecomastia.' Although obesity causes pseudo gynecomastia, which is a proliferation of fat rather than breast glandular tissue, true gynecomastia is also associated with higher body weight. Many studies, like ones by Rivera et al., indicated that there is a correlation between pubertal gynecomastia and higher BMI (Basal Metabolic Index) percentiles (Reference). Kulshreshtha et al. also reported that most of the patients (64 percent) with breast enlargement were obese as per scientific criteria (Reference).

WHAT IS BMI?

It is an anthropometric index of weight and height that is defined as:

Body weight in kilograms divided by height in metres squared (Keys et al., 1972).

BMI = weight (kg)/height (m)^2

BMI is the commonly accepted index for classifying adiposity in adults and it is recommended for use with children and adolescents. This useful measurement is used to identify individuals who are underweight or overweight. BMI is *not* a diagnostic tool (Barlow and Dietz, 1998).

For example, a relatively heavy child may have a high BMI for his or her age or high weight-for-stature. To ascertain whether the child has excess fat, a further assessment would be needed and that might include skinfold calipers measurements etc. For children, BMI is gender-specific and age-specific because BMI changes substantially as children get older. BMI-for-age is the measure used for children ages two to 20 years.

This is illustrated in the chart below:

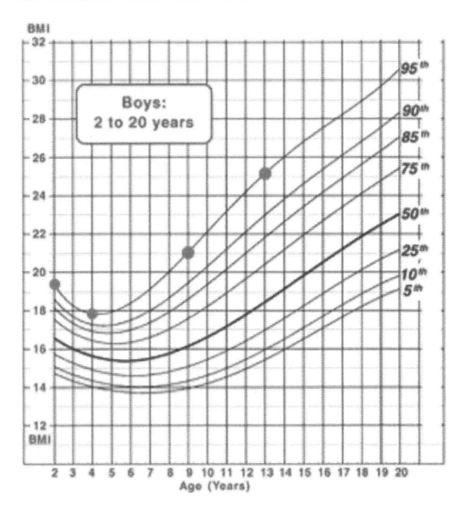

As illustrated on this growth chart for boys, in a growth pattern established along with the 95th percentile, BMI-for-age reached a minimum at four years of age and then increased with age.

RECOMMENDED BMI-FOR-AGE CUTOFFS

The expert committees' recommendations are to classify BMI-for-age at or above the 95th percentile as overweight and between the 85th and 95th percentile as at risk of being overweight.

"Overweight," rather than obesity, is the term preferred for describing children and adolescents with a BMI-for-age equal to or greater than the 95th percentile of BMI-for-age or weight-for-length.

The 85th percentile is included on the BMI-for-age and the weight-for-stature charts to identify those at risk of overweight.

This is different from the clinical guidelines established in 1998 by the National Heart, Lung and Blood Institute for adults as follows:

BMI less than 18.5 underweight

BMI of 18.5 through 24.9 normal

BMI of 25.0 through 29.9 overweight

BMI of 30.0 or greater obese

It is common to notice higher BMI values than the general population, according to the Centres for Disease Control (CDC) growth charts in gynecomastia patients. However, there is no relationship between BMI and breast size. Even though many overweight children (57.1 percent) succeed in losing some weight, breast size did not reduce in any of them and weight changes did not affect sex hormone levels. This observation—that weight loss alone will not correct actual glandular breast enlargement—is consistent with that reported by many other studies.

It should also be noted that, in the majority of our patients, the breasts do not show a drastic increase in size with age. Adolescents with gynecomastia should be encouraged to lose weight but it does not treat the underlying breast tissue.

Surgical management of pubertal gynecomastia may be considered in obese or non-obese male adolescents who present with persistent breast enlargement after a period of observation of at least 12 months, breast pain or tenderness and significant psycho-social distress. Obesity is not a contraindication to the surgical approach. Liposuction techniques are helpful in those patients with considerable fat deposition in the breast during the removal of the glandular component. Surgical treatment aims to achieve a normal appearance of the male thorax with the smallest possible scar. The surgical treatment of gynecomastia requires an individualised approach.

In conclusion, teenage boys who have persistent gynecomastia after the end of pubertal development, and adolescents who have concerns about the cosmetic correction can undergo gynecomastia surgery. Therefore, the decision to perform surgery depends on the degree to which this condition has affected the quality of life, psychology and the desire for cosmetic correction.

As for the maximum age for getting the gynecomastia surgery, the only criteria is the patient's medical fitness to undergo the procedure in the first place. There is no upper age limit.

Before one embarks upon gynecomastia surgery, both the surgeon and the patient should have an idea about what an ideal male chest is. The discussion makes sure everyone is clear what the male breast reduction surgery will achieve. Patients must understand that not every man can have the "ideal" chest. Various conditions—such as ageing, excess body weight, poor skin quality and unfavourable shape and anatomy—affect what is obtainable.

The first thing that one should understand is that the "ideal" chest is not flat. There is a defined contour, a slight bulge and a natural fold just below the chest where the abdomen begins. The chest fold is predominately horizontal. This horizontal line tends to round out and increases with the varying degrees of gynecomastia.

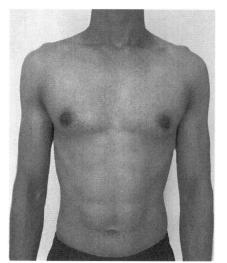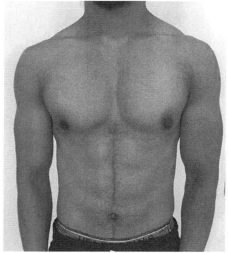

Different chests that men would consider ideal. Note the slight asymmetry in muscle angle and slight bulge.

On the "ideal" chest, the nipple is typically five to six centimetres above the chest fold and faces forward. But this differs according to the built of the patient and the race. The areola is flush with the surrounding skin. With certain types of gynecomastia, the areola will protrude forward, creating what is called "puffy nipple."

Even ideal male chests can have approximately a couple of centimetres of fat underneath. Since this is a natural part of the chest, it is not wise to completely remove all of the fat during surgery. Lastly, take a look at the contour/shape of the pectoralis major muscle in relation to the chest fold. It is the big muscle that gives the chest its muscular shape.

The "ideal" male chest may have some breast tissue located directly below the areola. You can feel it by squeezing the tissue under the areola. It is firm, glandular tissue, where fatty tissue is soft and squishy. This amount of breast tissue is sometimes considered normal. So, gynecomastia can be logically referred to as an excess of this normal breast tissue?

HEADING: SURGICAL STRATEGIES

Initially, the surgeries concentrated on removing the breast tissue like it was done in females. They would take out all the breast tissue through skin cuts that were not well-hidden and removed the entire gland that left behind a saucer-shaped contour deformity in many cases. A few unsatisfactory years later, many surgeons advocated only liposuction for grades one and two of gynecomastia. They never removed the gland. Over long-term follow-ups, they noticed that the breast gland appeared like a projecting blob under the nipple and most patients were unsatisfied with the chest shape. They felt that removing the fat worsened the chest as the gland stood out even more without the fat to smoothen its edges a little. This observation marked a paradigm shift in thinking and after a few more techniques came to fore, Teimourian and Pearlman described a combination of liposuction and removal of the gland for treating gynecomastia. This combination has now stood the test of time.

The skin incisions (cuts) have evolved over a period of time. Different incisions (skin cuts) have also been used. It is very important to choose and execute the right incision. I have had referrals of patients who underwent a surgery which was done through poorly planned incisions. Now their main issue would be an oddly placed scar more than the gynecomastia itself.

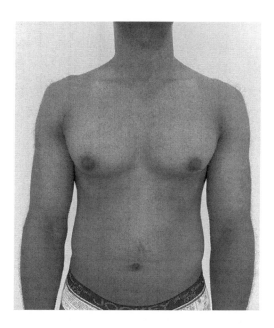

This man underwent surgery in a place where gynecomastia is not done commonly. The incisions were placed well below the areola leading to very visible and oddly placed obvious scars, especially on the left side.

Some of the incisions are described below:

1. Inferior circum-areolar incision: This is probably the most commonly used incision (skin cut) while approaching the breast gland.

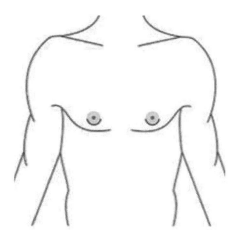

2. Intra-areolar incision, or Webster incision: Here, the cut extends along the circumference of the areola in the dark and pigmented portion. While the scar tends to be well-hidden in lighter skin types, even a minor irregularity or loss of skin pigment during healing leaves a more visible scar in coloured individuals. The length of the incision also varies according to the shape of the patient.

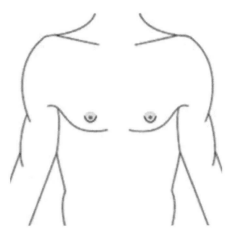

3. A cut along the lower circumference of the areola with lateral and medial extensions is another variation of the conventional circum-areolar incision. Though this incision makes the surgery more accessible, it is not commonly used due to its unnecessarily excess scarring.

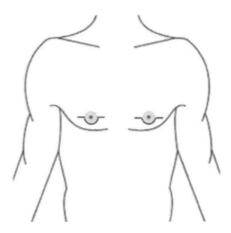

4. An incision that lies horizontally at the level of the nipple is a very rarely used one. Not only does it have the disadvantages of the first incision, but it also tended to change the shape of the nipple and hence is used very infrequently.

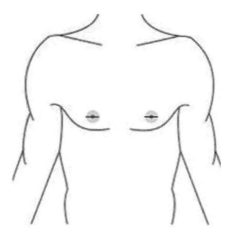

5. Elliptical incision: Here, the skin is cut in a transverse ellipse and the skin along with the breast tissue is removed in one block. It, however, requires placing the nipple and areola as a free graft (the nipple and areola are separated and then again put back at completion of the surgery). This incision is an option in large glands but has the drawback of visible scars and an uneven colour once healed.

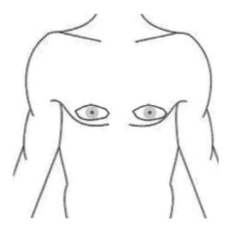

6. Triple V incision: This is used when the nipple and areola positions need to be repositioned in the same stage as removal of the gland. It has a few applications though it may be useful in one-sided gynecomastia to achieve better symmetry.

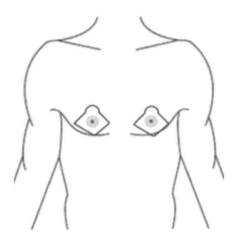

7. Armpit incision: Also called the axillary technique. This incision is an excellent option to hide the scar. But achieving a perfect symmetry is challenging with this approach.

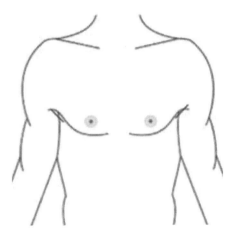

8. Other skin removal cuts and approaches: Many other incisions try to tackle the loose skin and breast tissue in the same sitting.

The shape and extent of these skin cuts depend on the amount and direction of loose skin. While they may leave large unsightly scars, they may be the only option in vary large grade three gynecomastia, especially when the patient wants to do it all in one sitting.

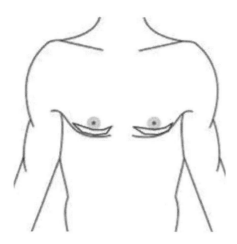

9. Small, minimally invasive techniques: These methods try to use smaller incisions than conventional techniques. Sometimes, even endoscopes are used to remove the glands. While this approach is enticing due to its reduced scarring, a pragmatic view is needed to balance the effort and surgical time required against reducing the scar by one centimetre. However, many surgeons are trying these techniques and such techniques may get more refined with time.

As the techniques got refined, many surgeons advocated only liposuction for grades one and two of gynecomastia. They never used to remove the gland. On long-term follow-ups, they noticed that the gland appeared like a projecting blob under the nipple and most patients were unsatisfied with the chest shape. They felt that removing the fat worsened the chest as the gland stood out even more without the fat to smoothen its edges a little. After the paradigm shift in thinking, Teimourian and Pearlman came up with the idea of combining the two. It was named differently and the commonest was 'lipo-excision'.

Since then, a combination of liposuction and removal of the gland has been in vogue for treating gynecomastia. However, this seemingly simple combination was far from refined and has gone through its fair share of changes and experiments. The hot topic of debate was how one should balance these two procedures. The other dilemmas were:

1. Is aggressive liposuction needed even in skinny-grade I patients?
2. Should liposuction be done through the same incision through which the gland would be removed, or does it need a separate incision?
3. What kind of liposuction is optimally suited?
4. Should the gland be removed in its entirety?
5. If the gland should not be removed completely, how much of it should be left behind?
6. How would combining both the procedures into one impact recovery and results?

These were just some of the questions the early surgeons had to answer. However, the answer was different among surgeons and very different depending on the race of the individual they operated upon, among other factors. I noticed that the European and, to an extent, American surgeons were happy leaving behind almost none of the gland, while Asian surgeons tended to leave more behind. There could be many reasons why there was such a gross difference in the techniques, though technically both were lipo-excision.

Okay, now let's discuss these questions one by one.

1. Ever since the combination of liposuction and excision of glands came at the forefront for treating gynecomastia, it has been used in all but very skinny or very muscular patients. Such patients, though uncommon, are not rare. In such individuals, there may not be enough fat that needs removing. A simple excision (complete or near-complete) would suffice. Such cases may occasionally be tricky in terms of the extent of gland removal. While complete removal is theoretically safe, it does lead to a subtle crater deformity. There is an argument for leaving a very thin sliver of gland behind in most people. Also, the merits of subtle liposuction to smoothen out the edges cannot be overstated. The expertise of a surgeon will, in most cases, determine the outcome. It is more challenging to treat such individuals than normally built men.

2. Once the decision to do both liposuction and gland excision is made, the next decision the surgeon and the patient, to an extent, face is the incision through which liposuction needs to be done. While it is generally agreed that excision is better through peri-areolar or intra-areolar incisions, the liposuction incision is more hotly debated and also varies widely in terms of the surgeon's preference. Many surgeons use an incision on the lower and lateral (to the side) part of the chest for liposuction. The main reason is that liposuction becomes very easy as the fat—especially the one below the areola—is easily accessible. This, however, comes at the price of an additional scar. While this scar may not be noticeable in fairer individuals, it is quite evident in darker-skinned men like most Indians. The advantage of doing liposuction through the same area where we would be cutting the skin for gland removal is that there is only one scar at the end of the procedure. The slight disadvantage is that the surgeon will find it a little tricky to remove the fat under the

areola. But this is something that can be overcome by practice. This is especially true as plastic surgeons are used to removing fat that is close to the incisions, like for a double chin. Hence, access to fat is not a strong enough reason to make an additional cut, in my opinion.

3. The first liposuctions that were done were called 'dry liposuctions.' Here, the surgeon just inserted a cannula into the area and sucked out the fat with a vacuum device. The main issues were the delayed recovery, difficulty in removing the fat evenly and excess bleeding during the procedure. The unacceptable downtime prompted surgeons to inject saline in varying quantities into the areas to be liposuctioned. These were called 'wet', 'super-wet' and 'tumescent' techniques depending on the amount of saline that was injected. These techniques quickly became the gold standard and are followed even today. Most follow either the super-wet or tumescent methods. Such infiltration allows the surgeon to minimise bleeding, do liposuction to more areas at once and achieve a better overall shape. The addition of a local anaesthetic solution to the saline further added the advantage that many regions of fat could be removed under local anaesthesia, thus negating the need for admission. But liposuction under local anaesthesia leads to other issues. One, the amount of aesthetic needed to anesthetise broad chests borders the permitted upper limit of dosage of local anaesthetic. Hence, the safety is frequently an issue. Two, the process of injecting such fluids to anesthetise the chest in the first place is quite painful, primarily until the aesthetic kicks in. Third, since the local anaesthetic has to be diluted for wider areas, the painlessness after injection is not as durable and, frequently, the patient is in discomfort, which again prompts the surgeon to either inject more aesthetic or do sub-optimal liposuction.

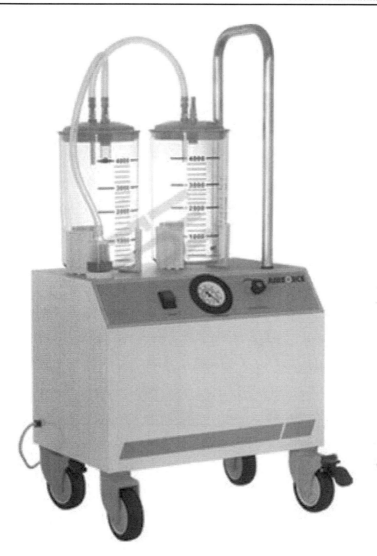

A regular liposuction machine

Apart from this classical method, there are many newer techniques. Power-assisted liposuction is a method wherein a power machine makes the cannula move front and back (or in a circle, in some cases), thus making the procedure faster with less effort from the surgeon. Results are, for the most part, similar to the classical techniques.

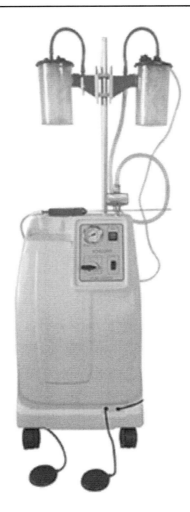

Power-assisted Liposuction machines

Ultrasonic liposuction (VASER, Lysonix, etc.) is a technique where the fat is liquefied using ultrasound mechanisms. The advantage is that it can be more precise while removing fat and, in turn, causes fewer traumas to the native tissues. But, in inexperienced hands, it has occasionally led to skin burns, especially at the entry points. However, this is a valuable addition to the armamentarium of a liposuction surgeon.

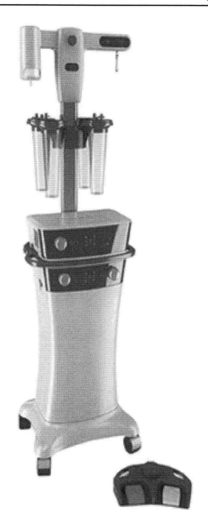

An Ultrasonic liposuction machine

Laser liposuction is the newer technique where a variety of lasers are used to liquefy and aspirate the fat. FDA (Food and Drug Administration of the USA) has approved the use of Nd-Yag and Diode lasers for laser lipolysis. The advantage over the classical techniques is a lesser downtime, smoother recovery, and better skin tightening.

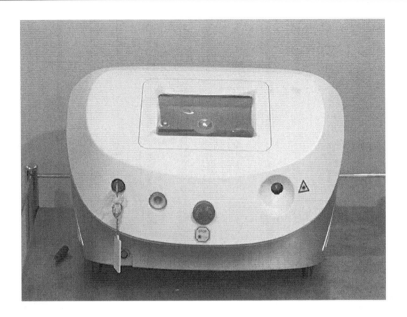

Laser liposuction machine

The new techniques are not without their drawbacks. There is a steeper learning curve with these techniques, unlike the classical methods. In medical schools, the classic methods are taught beforehand so that the surgeon is well-versed with the underlying mechanisms before using these more advanced instruments. The chances of skin burns are slightly high, especially in the initial period of the surgeon's learning. These also tend to make the procedure slower as compared to the classical technique. Lastly, they tend to be expensive machines to buy and maintain and, hence, the procedures done using them also tend to be proportionately more expensive.

All said and done, the choice of the technique of liposuction rests with the surgeon and the method he is most comfortable with. Over a period of time, surgeons generally tend to prefer one single method and are able to achieve consistent results with the one they use most often.

4. Removing the whole gland is standard practice with many surgeons across the world. The surgery is also commonly referred

to as a subcutaneous mastectomy. It means that the entire gland is removed. As highlighted by many surgeons over many years, this complete removal has a very high chance of leaving behind a depressed area under the areola, commonly called the 'crater deformity'. Such craters are seen in many individuals though, occasionally, the surgeon may feel no need to leave anything behind and still achieve a perfect shape. Such exceptions are made after taking into account factors like the size and bulkiness of the chest muscles, fat distribution over the chest and skin tone, among others.

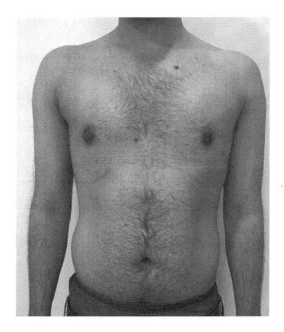

Notice the subtle crater deformity after overzealous removal of the entire breast. Deeper and worse 'craters' are not unknown

5. Once the surgical planning involves leaving a certain amount of breast tissue behind, the next question is just how much of it needs to be left behind? Many earlier advocates of such techniques recommended leaving behind a disc of breast tissue about three centimetres in diameter and about one centimetre

thick under the areola. While this guideline can be accurate in some cases, this by no means can be a general guideline. The amount of tissue that needs to be left behind obviously depends on the chest size, amount of breast tissue, amount of looseness of skin, the patient's general fat distribution and thickness of fat adjacent to breast tissue, size of his chest muscle, age of the patient and his likelihood of maintaining a certain fitness levels. Now, when there are so many factors that can predict the amount of breast tissue that, when left behind, would suit a person, it is highly unlikely that a standard guideline can be put forward to all patients. I have left behind tissue ranging from nil to a 12-centimetre disc of tissue. Even the thickness can vary from nil to two or three centimetres. When there is such a wide variation, the judgement depends solely on the surgeon who is best placed to assess all of the above factors during the surgery. Though he may proceed with a pre-surgical plan of a certain amount of tissue to leave behind, that may change once liposuction and initial tissue dissection is complete.

Another critical issue is how the tissue that you leave behind survives there. Like any part of the body, even the breast tissue needs blood supply to survive. To make sure that the blood supply stays intact, it needs to be attached to the areas where its blood supply is likely to come from. Usually, the tissue survives entirely when it is attached to the skin under the areola (as was done earlier) or when it's attached superiorly (upper part of the breast) where its actual blood supply is coming from. It is to be noted that the breast gets its blood from various blood vessels. The most important comes from the intercostal vessels (the ones that run between the ribs). The most vital of them come from the second to forth intercostal vessels and traverse for the superior direction (meaning come from the upper chest downwards). Hence, there is logic in not only leaving tissue behind, but also keeping it attached in a particular direction to preserve the blood supply.

6. While it is evident that lipo-excision is more invasive than either one of the procedures alone, it is, however, necessary for all the reasons discussed above. The recovery is a bit more painful and the bruising and swelling proportionately more when two procedures are combined as one. But that is what an adequate gynecomastia correction demands.

Chapter 5

DECISION-MAKING AND CONSENT

The decision of whether to undergo surgery is entirely the patient's. The first thing one needs to understand is that gynecomastia is purely cosmetic surgery and hence is not compulsory. It is worthwhile reading up the surgical decision-making protocol, as suggested by the Hopkin's institute. While this is a general guideline for any surgery, it applies to gynecomastia surgery as well. It's as below:

CHECKLIST FOR SURGERY

The decision to have surgery is a significant one. You will need to be fully informed and prepared for the operation. You will also need to be ready for any special needs that you may have after the surgery. How well you prepare will affect the outcome and the results. The following is a checklist to help you get ready for surgery:

1. Make a list of questions to ask your healthcare provider or surgeon about the type of surgery you are to have.

2. Talk with your provider to find out if the surgery is right for you.

3. Get a second opinion if you want to.

4. Check with your health plan about what costs of the surgery you will be responsible for. In most cases, gynecomastia is not covered by insurance.

5. Get a list of costs from your doctors and the hospital or outpatient facility.

6. Schedule the surgery.

7. Make a list of all the medicines you take. The list includes all prescription and over-the-counter drugs, and all herbal supplements. Go over this list with the anaesthesiologist and surgeons.

8. Schedule any lab tests you need to have before the surgery.

9. Set up a meeting with the anaesthesiologist before the surgery if necessary.

10. Follow all instructions during the weeks and days before the surgery.

11. Stop taking any medicines or supplements that your surgeon tells you to before the surgery.

12. Arrange for any home care or equipment you will need at home after the surgery.

13. Sign all informed consent and other legal forms before surgery after reading and understanding them.

14. Quit smoking several weeks before the surgery. It will help you recover faster. It will also help your incision heal more quickly.

15. Remove all jewellery and metal objects before the surgery.

CONSENT FOR SURGERY AND ANAESTHESIA

A patient's (or attender's/surrogate's) informed consent generally is required before diagnostic and treatment interventions, except in cases of minors, emergencies, threats to public health, danger to self or others or any special exceptions. A consent form is necessary before a gynecomastia surgery can be done.

The patient needs to read, understand and sign the consent before the surgery. He also needs to clear any doubts about the surgery, anaesthesia or the consent form with the surgeon and anaesthetist before the procedure starts. The forms should be signed on by the patient on every page.

The purposes of consent forms are:

1. To help the patient better understand the procedure objectively.

2. It is another chance for the patient to clarify any doubts and ask the surgeon/anaesthetist questions about the procedure.

3. It is also a legal document that the patient agrees to undergo surgery after understanding the relevant risks.

4. Build trust between the patient and the surgical team. It clears up doubts more objectively.

These are the consent forms we use at our clinic:

GYNECOMASTIA SURGERY-CONSENT FORM

1. I authorise the performance on (Name of patient) _____ the lipo-excision surgery to be performed by, or under the direction of, Dr Sreekar Harinatha together with associates or assistants of his choice who may be employed by the him.

2. The doctor has discussed the procedure with me and I understand the following items:

   A. The nature and purpose of the proposed procedure(s).

   B. The risks of the proposed procedure(s).

   C. The possible or likely consequences of the proposed procedure(s).

   D. All available or alternative treatments (including the risks, consequences and probable effectiveness).

3. I consent to the performance of operation(s) and procedure(s) in addition to or those different from those now contemplated, arising from presently unforeseen conditions, which the above-

named doctor or his associates or assistants may consider necessary or advisable in emergency or life-threatening situations.

4. I acknowledge that no guarantee or assurance has been given by anyone as to the results that may be obtained.

5. I understand that the physicians, anaesthesiologists and nursing staff who participate in the surgery are independent professionals and are not permanent employees of the clinic.

6. My consent is given with the understanding that any operation or procedure, including anaesthesia, involves risks and hazards. The more common risks include (but are not limited to) infection, bleeding requiring blood transfusion(s), nerve injury, blood clots, heart attack, stroke, allergic reaction(s), damage to teeth or bridgework and pneumonia. These risks can be severe and possibly fatal.

7. I consent to the performance of operations or other procedures in addition to or different from those now contemplated whether or not arising from presently unforeseen conditions, including the implantation of medical devices which the above-named physician(s) or his/her associate(s) or assistant(s) may consider necessary or advisable in the course of the operation.

8. I understand the risks, benefits and alternatives to the type and method of anaesthesia or sedation recommended. I consent to the administration of such anaesthesia as may be considered necessary or advisable by the physician(s) for this surgery/procedure.

9. I consent to the photographing or videotaping before, after and of the surgery or procedure(s) to be performed, including appropriate portions of my body for medical, scientific or educational purposes, provided that my identity is not revealed by the pictures or by descriptive texts accompanying them.

10. I consent to the presence of observers in the operating room, such as students, medical residents, medical equipment representatives or other appropriate parties approved by my surgeon(s).

11. I consent to the disposal of any human tissue or body part which may be removed during the surgery/procedure (s).

12. If complications arise, I agree to be admitted to the hospital of my surgeon's choice.

13. I have been advised that there is a possibility of damage to teeth during surgery and administration of anaesthesia, particularly if the teeth are weak, loose, decayed or artificial, and I waive any claim for damage to teeth as a result thereof.

14. I understand that, unless instructed otherwise, I am required to have a responsible adult accompany me after my surgery/ procedure (s) and that I will be released to that person's custody and must rely upon him/her for my return home and supervision, as instructed.

15. I release the surgery centre from any responsibility for loss of or damage to money, jewellery or other valuables I have brought to the surgery centre.

16. I understand that if I am suffering from any known illnesses, I must inform the surgery centre immediately since this could lead to complications during the scheduled surgery/procedure(s).

17. If I am not the patient, I represent that I have the authority of the patient who, because of age or other legal disability, is unable to consent to the matters above. I represent that (a) I have the full right to consent to the matters above; (b) I agree to release, indemnify and hold harmless the surgery centre, its employees, agents, medical staff, partners and affiliates from any liability or cost arising out of my lack of adequate authority to provide the consent set forth herein.

18. I realise that, as in all medical treatments, complications or delays in recovery may occur, which could lead to the need for additional treatment or surgery and could also result in economic loss to me because of my inability to return to regular activity as soon as anticipated. I understand that, in the event of any revision surgery taking place for whatever reason, then, although the surgeon's fee may be waived in these circumstances, I will be responsible for any anaesthetists, hospital or theatre facility fee.

19. I understand that external incisions leave visible scars. The location of these incisions has been described to me. I also understand that it is impossible to predict the exact ultimate appearance of these scars despite meticulous technique. I have been advised that scars take upwards of 18 months to mature and the changes that generally occur in their appearance during the healing period, such as redness, lumpiness and irregularities, have been described to me. I also realise that although unsightly scars can be surgically revised, this does not provide any guarantee that the subsequent ensuing appearance of the scar will be invisible.

20. I understand that the practice of medicine and surgery is not an exact science and different people can react differently to one procedure. Further, the results vary in different people. I understand that this procedure is performed for cosmetic reasons and, because of this, the results can only be assessed subjectively. Therefore, I understand that, while I have been advised as to the probable outcome, this should in no way be interpreted as a guarantee. No explicit guarantees or assurance have been made to me concerning the results of this procedure. I fully understand that it is possible that the result might not live up to my expectations or the goals that may have been established by myself or the surgeon.

THE POSSIBLE RISKS INVOLVED WITH GYNECOMASTIA SURGERY

Gynecomastia surgery primarily consists of two parts: Liposuction and Excision.

Liposuction consists of removal of body fat by using a device called a cannula, which sucks fat cells and then completes the removal by suction. This procedure is effective in removing fat in different parts of the body like chest, abdomen, etc. It should be emphasised from the outset that the process has limitations in the amount of fat that can be removed and the amount of body sculpting that can be accomplished. However, in a patient in whom there is an abnormal deposition of fat, it is extremely helpful in removing some of this fat in order to enhance one's appearance.

The procedure is most effective in young patients with good skin elasticity, as the skin will contract after the fat has been removed. Where abnormal collections of fat have developed, it has been beneficial in recontouring the specific part.

In this procedure, liposuction is done to the chest to improve the contour.

Following liposuction, the breast tissue is removed (excised). In our method of gynecomastia surgery, we target sub-total removal of the gland (around 90 percent) to achieve a better contour. The amount left behind depends on the body shape, amount of fat and muscles in the area and surrounding it and is at the discretion of the operating surgeon.

COMPLICATIONS

As with any operation, certain problems can occur as a result of this procedure and it is vital that you are aware of the risks involved. Although permanent problems infrequently occur, complications that have been noted with this procedure include thickened or unattractive scars at the site of the small incisions used to introduce the suction device, irregularity of contour of the area treated and possibility of skin loss which may result in permanent scarring of the area or the need for skin grafting, wrinkling, sagging of the skin, numbness in the area treated, prolonged swelling and accumulation of blood or serum under the skin, requiring removal.

The immediate post-operative risks involved in this procedure are asymmetry, infection, seroma, hematoma, pain and pulmonary embolism (blood clot to lungs-rare), pulmonary fat embolism syndrome (fat in the lungs-extremely rare), tear of underlying muscle resulting in pain and rarely compartment syndrome, perforation of the pleura/perforation of the chest wall and its sequelae. There is also the possibility that you may not look better from this operation and it is conceivable that you may even look worse, should complications occur. This information is not provided to frighten or intimidate you but rather to acquaint you with the risks associated with this procedure so that if you elect to have such an operation, it is with an understanding of the complications that can occur. It is not possible to advise you of every conceivable complication and other problems can occur that are unexpected. The potential exists for personality changes such as profound depression after this operation. Let it be known that the risks associated with this procedure are directly related to the amount suctioned and the age of the patient.

The issues specific to excision surgery, especially temporary ones like serous discharge, hematoma, and numbness, etc. and permanent ones like-scars, nipple, or nipple-areola contour irregularity, asymmetry, permanent numbness, loose skin and the treatment of complications have been discussed in detail.

The reasons for the gynecomastia in most of the cases is unknown and the rare possibility of re-occurrence of the swelling has been explained to me. If any of these complications arise, the treatment has been explained to me. If any new complication may occur, which may not have been discussed, the treating surgeon, his team and this hospital will not be held responsible.

The complete disease, investigations required and different modalities of treatment have also been discussed with me in detail.

I HAVE READ THE INFORMED CONSENT FOR GYNECOMASTIA SURGERY AND POSSIBLE RISKS INVOLVED WITH THIS PROCEDURE.

MY SIGNATURE BELOW CONSTITUTES MY ACKNOWLEDGEMENT THAT:

1. I have read, understand and agree to the foregoing;
2. The proposed surgery/procedure(s) have been satisfactorily explained to me and that I have all of the information that I require;
3. I hereby give my authorisation and consent;
4. All blank spaces on this document have either been accepted and completed or crossed off if they do not apply before my signing;
5. I have read and fully understand this entire form. I have asked the doctor any questions I may have had, and the doctor has answered all my questions to my satisfaction.

Name	Signature	Date
Patient		
Witness		
Surgeon		

INFORMATION FOR CONSENT TO ANAESTHESIA

The purpose of this consent form is to inform you and your family about some of the possible risks of having anaesthesia.

1. Anaesthesia is needed to relieve you of pain and stress during surgical procedures. However, all forms of anaesthesia involve some risks, even death. The reported peri-operative mortality rate correlates with a patient's pre-operative health conditions. Classification system adopted by the American Society of Anaesthesiologists to classify patients into risk categories is as follows:

   Class1: normal healthy patient

   Class2: mild systemic disease and no functional limitations

   Class3: moderate to severe systemic disease that results in some functional limitations

   Class4: severe systemic disease that is a constant threat to life and functionally incapacitating

   Class5: not expected to survive 24 h with or without surgery

2. As with any other medical intervention, there are risks of potential complications with virtually all forms of anaesthesia.

   A. Existing or past medical problems may add risk during and after surgery.

      i. Cardiovascular problems such as angina, a previous heart attack, heart failure, hypertension or valvular heart disease increase your risk of myocardial infarction and stroke.

      ii. Lung problems such as asthma, respiratory tract infection or chronic obstructive pulmonary disorders may worsen your lung condition after surgery.

  iii. Other conditions such as liver disease, kidney problems, endocrine disorders, cancer, alcohol or drug abuse also increase your risk.

  iv. The anaesthesiologist providing your care is a skilled specialist who is trained to foresee and prevent most of the problems.

Some critical problems occurring during or after anaesthesia may mandate for you to stay in the intensive care unit after surgery.

  B. During anaesthesia, we must keep your airway open using a small tube (endotracheal tube or laryngeal mask airway). These tubes can rarely result in injury to your teeth, dental work, tongue, lips, nose or throat. You may have a sore throat from the airway used during surgery.

  C. You may vomit the contents of your stomach during surgery. They may enter the lungs and cause breathing problems. This risk of aspiration will significantly increase in emergency surgery or a patient with increased abdominal pressure (intestinal obstruction or pregnancy).

  D. You may have adverse reactions to drugs or blood products you receive during surgery. On rare occasions, these may be life-threatening.

  E. You may sometimes have skin or nerve injury from positioning required for surgery or equipment used during surgery.

  F. You may have a headache after anaesthesia. On rare occasions, transient neurological symptoms or even permanent nerve damage can occur.

  G. Some drugs given during surgery may cause your muscles to be sore and stiff.

  H. Although rarely occurs, an incidence of 0.2 percent is reported for the occurrence of awareness during general anaesthesia.

Most of these cases are reported by patients undergoing major cardiothoracic surgeries.

I. Although, rarely, malignant hyperthermia may occur in genetically susceptible patients after exposure to an anaesthetic triggering agent (1:15,000 in paediatric patients and 1:40,000 in adult patients).

J. While waking up from anaesthesia, some patients may shake or shiver.

K. Some patients feel nauseated or vomit after surgery or anaesthesia. This can be influenced by a history of motion sickness, the type of surgery performed, anaesthetics used during surgery and the pain medications after surgery.

3. In the event of a sudden unexpected critical condition (hypoxic brain injury or massive bleeding), extraordinary measures (surgical tracheostomy to secure the airway or arterial and central venous catheter insertion to stabilise circulation) may become necessary.

4. If you still have questions about any part of the intraoperative events or anaesthetic plans, please talk to your doctor or anaesthesiologist about them before surgery.

PATIENT'S ACKNOWLEDGEMENT

A. I understand that anaesthesia services are necessary for surgical treatment.

B. My anaesthesiologist has explained the anaesthetic procedures and their risks to me and I had ample time to ask questions and to consider my decision.

C. I have also read the **"INFORMATION FOR CONSENT TO ANAESTHESIA"** form and understand the risks of the anaesthetic procedures.

I hereby consent to the anaesthetic procedures checked above.

Name	Signature	Date
Patient		
Witness		
Surgeon		
Anaesthetist		

OUR TECHNIQUE

We follow the modified superior dynamic flap method. Let us understand the name first. It is 'superior' because the blood supply coming to the tissue from the superior direction is intact and 'dynamic' because of the distribution and amount of the tissue that can be adjusted for a better overall shape. 'Flap' is a tissue that is transferred from one place to another with its blood supply intact—in this case, the 'breast tissue.'

PRE-PROCEDURE PREPARATION

The essential aspects of surgery start before the surgery itself. The pre-surgical markings are made in the pre-operative holding area with the patient standing. This is a vital part of planning as accurate planning can note down different factors and issues:

1. Amount and distribution of fat over the chest

2. Amount and distribution of the breast tissue

3. The asymmetry between the two sides-In terms of fat, breast, nipple, and areola

4. Assessment of skin laxity and tone

5. Any other issue that may affect surgical results

The extent of the chest bulges is marked first. The first markings are of the areas of excess fat that needs to be treated along with the breast tissue. This mark continues to the inframammary fold (Fold under the breast tissue). This mark forms the outer boundary of the surgical area. Then, the palpable breast gland is marked. To facilitate easier isolation of the gland, the chest (pectoral) muscles are contracted by asking the patient to press the hips with his arms. Once the muscle is taught, the gland stands out for easier marking. Next, the glandular markings are confirmed by asking the patient to raise his arms while the breast tissue is held by the surgeon's fingers. This is repeated on the other side. Also important to mark are the chest skin folds, especially on the sides. They too need to be treated effectively for a better contour.

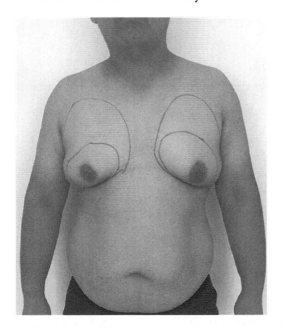

The outer markings are the areas of fat that need to be treated.
The inner marking is of the boundaries of the breast gland.

ANAESTHESIA

The word anaesthesia evokes mixed feelings among many people. This is wholly due the undue wrong press it gets in mainstream media. Anyway, gynecomastia can be done under local (with or without added sedation) or general anaesthesia. Local anaesthesia is one where the aesthetic solution is injected into the operating area (chest in this case) while in general anaesthesia you literally fall asleep and get up after the effect is reversed.

There are advantages and disadvantages of both. The advantages of local anaesthesia for gynecomastia are:

1. The recovery is generally faster as there is no or minimal sedation.

2. Post-procedure nausea and vomiting is uncommon.

3. Not many work-up investigations are generally needed.

4. Can be administered by the surgeon himself.

5. Cheaper than general anaesthesia.

DISADVANTAGES ARE:

1. The pain while injecting the aesthetic solution may be unbearable in many. As the area and amount of solution to anesthetise the chest is wide.

2. Sometimes, when the procedure becomes intolerable, another one may need to be scheduled to complete the surgery.

3. The amount of local anaesthetic needed is quite high. To circumvent this, many surgeons dilute it to an extent that it may be less effective

GENERAL ANAESTHESIA IS WHAT IS COMMONLY PREFERRED BY MANY SURGEONS. THE ADVANTAGES ARE:

1. The procedure itself is quite smooth.

2. The anaesthetist is always at hand to take care of any eventualities.

3. With the newer aesthetic drugs, the recovery also tends to be faster thus facilitating a day care discharge.

THE DISADVANTAGES ARE:

1. Post-procedure nausea and vomiting may be an issue in certain cases.

2. An obvious longer stay than a local anaesthesia procedure.

3. The overall costs tend to be higher.

IN THE OPERATING ROOM

The patients are given general anaesthesia and positioned supine (lying face upwards) with the arms abducted (arms at right angles). A hypotensive (the pressure is maintained slightly low) anaesthesia is paramount to a bloodless field for dissection and for minimising blood loss. First, we start with liposuction through a small incision at the lower part of the areola and infiltrations of wetting solution performed. The infiltrate solution contains one ampoule of 1:1,000 adrenaline in one litre of lactated ringer solution. Some amount of adrenaline is added to again reduce the blood loss. Liposuction is performed with a suction machine. The machine creates negative pressure and pulls out the liquefied fat through the cannula. This is facilitated by the to-and-fro movement of the cannula by the surgeon. The surgeon's experience comes in handy for a smooth, even and symmetric liposuction. Over-doing or under-doing it may affect the final shape.

The focus is also on reducing the fat folds over the chest, and smoothening out the whole of the chest wall in accordance to the final shape. The liposuction also helps in creation of a bloodless dissecting field and isolates the gland to a great extent making dissection simpler. The amount of fat aspirated is recorded and compared to the opposite side. This amount may not necessarily be same between the two sides. In fact, it's rarely ever the same. The liposuction also proceeds through the gland onto the lateral areas. Once the liposuction is completed, the gland dissection is started.

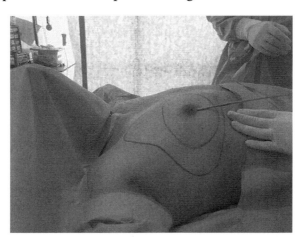

Liposuction is being done through the same area where the incision for gland removal will be done.

An inferior peri-areolar incision is then made and dissection proceeds all around the 360 degrees. This skin cut is around two to three centimetres long along the border of the areolar dark skin. What makes the eventual scar less obvious is its location in between the darker areolar skin and the surrounding fairer skin.

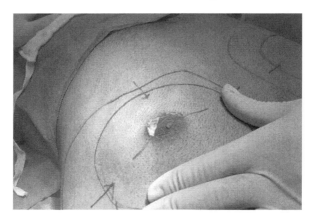

The inferior circum-areolar incision is done and the dissection is started.

The initial plane of dissection is along the subcutaneous (in the fat player under the skin) plane. Initially, the assistant raises the areola with skin hooks and the plane is dissected between the breast and the subcutaneous tissue. This extends all around until the skin with its fat is almost raised off of the gland. Then, the gland is elevated from the pectoral fascia (the thin layer of fascia covering the chest muscle—pectoralis major muscle) starting inferiorly (from the lower part of the gland). The gland is elevated from all sides except for the superior aspect from where the blood supply to the gland remains intact. Thus, the gland is elevated a superior based vascular flap (meaning, the breast tissue is elevated with its blood supply intact). The gland is externalised and the amount of depression it created on the chest is assessed.

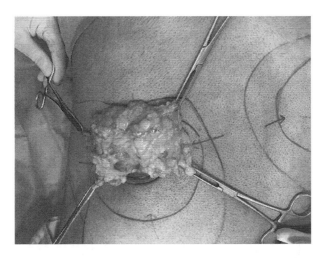

The exteriorised gland with its blood supply intact

Also, the amount of any irregularities on the chest wall are assessed and marked. Then, the gland is held taut and the excess gland is excised while saving the necessary amount to compensate for the contour irregularities. This remaining gland normally amounts to between five to 20 percent of the dissected tissue. The amount also depends on the overall patient contour, amount of fat, size of the pectoral muscles and the amount of asymmetry between the either sides that needs to be corrected.

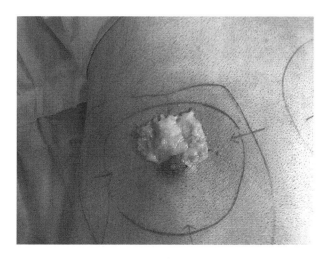

The trimmed gland that will be put back to achieve a better contour.

The remaining tissue is then inserted back through the incision and sutured to the pectorals major muscle with absorbable 3-0 sutures all around. As the vascularity of the glandular tissue is intact, the healing is usually smooth. Also, the direction and extent of pull during fixation can be adjusted depending on the location of correction that is needed. After this, the symmetry and overall shape is checked and stitches are put for the incision. Additionally, small adhesive paper strips called Stere-Strips are used to support the wound healing. A compression dressing is done to close the dissection spaces and reduce the chances of collection (seroma).

Many surgeons insert small pipes that are attached to a plastic bag to take out any remaining fluid. These are called drains. We have not felt the need to use them as the bleeding points are well controlled. Another issue with using the drains is that it is quite painful and it leave behind scars at the area where it is inserted.

Following the surgery, a compression dressing is done with elastic bandages which are removed after two days. Following this, a compression vest was advised for six weeks. The surgical video is available at *https://youtu.be/liXlcLOWqi4* or you can scan the QR code:

The surgery is invariably done on a day care basis. Occasionally, the surgeon may advise overnight admission due to the following reasons:

1. Delay in the surgery due to a late start or extended duration of the surgery itself.

2. If the surgeon or anaesthetist notices something unusual that may warrant monitoring. For example, poor breathing effort, excessive chest swelling, excess drowsiness, etc.

3. If gynecomastia is combined with other procedures, like liposuction, etc.

4. If the patient himself wants to be checked out the next day.

Chapter 6

POST-PROCEDURE INSTRUCTIONS

1. Diet: Regular diet—Avoid fat, alcohol or too much salt.
2. Smoking delays wound healing significantly and hence is better avoided for at least a few months after the surgery.
3. It is advised to use a pillow while sleeping for the first 48-72 hours. This is to help decrease swelling and for comfort. Avoid lying flat.
4. The dressing over the chest is removed after two to three days and the patient can shower after that. Use warm water when showering. Make sure there is someone with the patient the first time they shower in case they start to feel light-headed.
5. The surgical garment is to be worn for 23 hours a day for at least six weeks. It may be taken off while showering.
6. An antiseptic ointment is applied to the suture line twice daily after cleaning with soap and water. The area is covered with a gauze and micropore tape and then the pressure garment is worn.
7. The steri-strips are left in place after the first dressing and are removed or will fall off in five to seven days.
8. No lifting anything heavier than two to three kilograms or increasing heart rate for at least three weeks after surgery. No exercise until cleared.
9. Avoid riding a bike or driving for at least two weeks.

10. Avoid lifting your hand over-head for three weeks.

11. The patient can resume your full workouts only after three weeks. In the meanwhile, light exercises like walking for the lower part of your body can be done. Again, vigorous workouts are avoided.

12. While getting up from bed; the patient is to turn to one side and get up slowly. He should avoid pressing-down with hands as it may stretch the muscles in shoulder and chest.

13. Avoid wearing round neck T-shirts for two weeks.

COMPRESSION GARMENT

A compression garment after gynecomastia surgery is mandatory. It serves many purposes:

1. It helps reduce the swelling over the chest faster.

2. It helps the excess skin if any shrink faster.

3. It helps the overall skin reshaping to be smoother.

4. The constant pressure of the garment helps prevent any collection in the operated cavity.

5. It will help the patient achieve the final result faster.

When the patient wakes up from your procedure, he may already have a compression dressing on or may have a large dressing on the chest. Some surgeons prefer to put the pressure garment during the first dressing while some do it immediately after the surgery. Both are acceptable methods for compression.

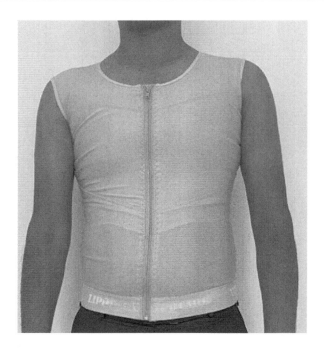

A tight compression garment is very important for prompt recovery

The garments may be made of linen, lycra and other materials. The preference lies with the patient. An important care regarding the garment is to avoid wringing it while washing as it tends to lose its elasticity by doing that. As the patient wears the garment, it tends to become loose both due to loss of its elasticity and due to reduction in the swelling on the chest. It is advisable to get it tightened and continue wearing it for the prescribed period. A loose garment is as good as not wearing one.

POST-SURGERY RECOVERY

After the surgery, the patients tend to be drowsy for a while until the full effect of the sedatives wear off. Then, gradually, the patient is allowed liquids first before he can eat. This may take a few hours. Drinking fluids too early may induce vomiting. Once the patient has had something to drink, he is encouraged to sit up with support before he stands and walks. Importantly, while sitting up, it is best to avoid pulling himself straight up especially by holding the cot or the side rails of the cot. This may put excess pressure and traction on the operated area and cause swelling. It's always better to turn on the bed to one side and then sit up using the side muscles. If he is not feeling drowsy or nauseous, he can slowly stand with support. Once he stands, he is advised to stay put for a few seconds before he walks. Doing all these quickly may cause light headedness. The doctor will check on the patient again before he is discharged.

The criteria for a safe discharge are:

1. Patient is awake, alert, responds to commands appropriate to age or returns to pre-procedure status.

2. Oxygen saturation (SpO2) greater than 95 percent or pre-procedure baseline on room air for 30 minutes without airway support.

3. Breathing is even and unlaboured.

4. Respiratory rate greater than 10 and less than 30 for adults.

5. Patient is able to sit in an upright position without signs and symptoms of orthostatic hypotension or light headedness.

6. The blood pressure is +/- 20 Hg mm of pre-procedure range or within patient's stated normal range.

7. No active bleeding or significant swelling at the operated site.

8. He is able to walk with minimal assistance or at pre-procedure level.

9. Tolerable pain: Pain score at rest is < 4 or at pre-procedure level at rest and patient states adequate pain control.

10. No IV opioids or sedatives given within 30 minutes.

11. Patient is not actively vomiting and nausea is mild in severity.

12. Patient is able to void (pass urine).

13. Intravenous injections and saline are completed as per post-procedure instructions.

14. Arrangements have been confirmed for a responsible adult to accompany the patient home and an individual remains available for the first 24 hours.

15. Discharge medication prescriptions are given to the patient.

16. Patient discharge teaching and written instructions are provided to the attender.

17. Blood sugar levels are controlled.

INSTRUCTIONS TO BE FOLLOWED AT HOME BEFORE THE FOLLOW-UP

The post-procedure check-up is normally scheduled after two to three days of the surgery. The patient is required to follow a few instructions in the meantime:

1. The patient can shower if he can avoid wetting the dressing on the chest. A towel bath is easier.

2. He can eat a normal diet that he is used to. A balanced diet is a must for optimal healing.

3. It is always better to have a friend or a relative along with the patient if the need arises.

4. The patient and relatives are given the numbers they can contact in case of emergencies, like bleeding from the operated site, breathlessness, light headedness, seizures etc.

5. In such emergency situations, the patient may need to visit the hospital again.

6. The patient is expected to follow the discharge instructions as listed on the discharge summary and as explained by the hospital staff.

7. The patient should avoid lifting heavy weight and avoid ding any sudden movements with the shoulders. Doing so may lead to collection or swelling over the operated area.

THE FOLLOW-UP VISIT

The follow-up visit after the surgery is normally scheduled after two or three days. During the visit, the surgeon will take out the dressing over the patient's chest and examine. He will check for any signs of collection, status of the stitches and whether the healing is optimal. It is quite common to notice bruising over the chest especially on the sides. This is normal and will subside in a week or two. It is also normal to feel a little tender when the operated areas are touched. Some areas will also feel numb.

If the surgeon notices a significant amount of collection/seroma, he may decide to aspirate it. This procedure will involve taking a few injections through which the collected fluid is sucked out. Sometimes, the surgeon may even open a part of stitched area to evacuate the collection. Often, the collection may not be fully aspirated as it is in a semi-solid state. In such cases, a further visit may be scheduled after a few days to complete the aspiration. Once aspirated, compression over the chest is mandatory to avoid recollection. This may be in the form of a tight dressing, a compression vest or both.

After the examination of the chest, the surgeon will then proceed with further instructions about wound care, massage, use of pressure garments and other dos and don'ts.

Massage: One very important yet understated post-surgical advice is about the massage. Massage is advised starting three weeks after the surgery and may need to continue for six weeks to six months. The duration depends on the grade of gynecomastia. The main factors being the amount of skin laxity and skin tone. The purposes of massage are:

1. To help decrease the swelling faster.

2. To smooth out any minor irregularities.

3. Reduce the chances of fluid collection.

4. Reduce spasms of the underlying muscles.

Massage is done to stimulate and augment the natural action of the lymphatic system. The lymphatic system is one of the critical aspects of the reduction in post-procedure swelling. It is often not given its due importance. For effective lymphatic massage, it is necessary to massage and pump in a specific direction at a specific pace. Most of the steps advised below are a combination of UHN (University Health Network) and Vodder School guidelines.

The massage has two parts:

– Steps to stimulate and activate the local lymphatic system.

– Steps to reduce chest swelling through chest massage.

Steps to stimulate and activate the local lymphatic system:

1. Deep breathing helps to boost the lymphatic system in the whole body. The steps are:

   • Place the palms or flats of your hands on your stomach.

   • Slowly, breathe in deeply through your nose, and let your stomach expand.

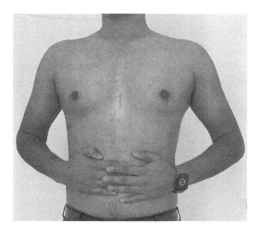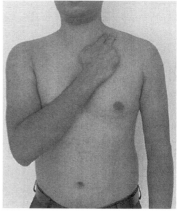

- Breathe out slowly through pursed lips (as if you were about to blow out a candle), and let your stomach flatten.

- Repeat five times. Take a short rest between each breath so you do not get dizzy.

2. Stretch and release the skin at the front of your neck. This step helps lymph fluid drain back to your heart. You can massage one side at a time, or do both sides together by crossing your hands.

   - Place the flats of your 2nd and 3rd fingers on either side of your neck, just above your collarbone.

   - Massage down and inwards towards your collarbone. Always keep your fingers above your collarbone. Gently stretch the skin just as far as it naturally goes and release.

   - This massage will look like two "J" strokes facing one another.

   - Repeat 15 times.

3. Stretch and release the skin at the side of your neck. You can massage one side at a time, or do both sides together.

   - Place your flat hands on either side of your neck, just under your ears.

   - Gently stretch the skin back (away from your face) and down, then release.

   - Try to massage your neck in a slow, gentle way, following a rhythm.

   - Repeat 10 to 15 times.

Remember: Keep your pressure light and your hands soft and relaxed.

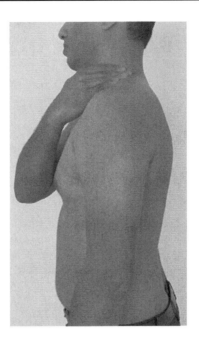

4. Stretch and release the skin on the back of your neck.

- Place your flat hands on the back of your neck, just below your hairline on either side of your spine.

- Stretch the skin towards your spine and then down towards the base of your neck and release.

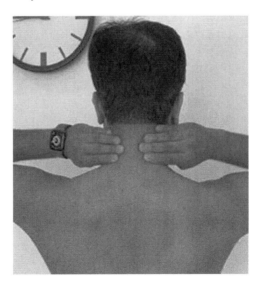

- Repeat 10 to 15 times.

Steps to reduce chest swelling through chest massage:

Lymphatic chest massage is reasonably easy to learn. A pumping movement is used wherein the chest is moved using some light pressure and then released, allowing it to return to the normal position.

Each move and return counts as one pump. In the lymphatic breast massage model, the most important idea is to keep the lymphatic fluid moving in this area.

Step 1: Put your hand in your armpit and push inward and upward. Go deep into the armpit. Pump upward and release. Do this ten to 20 times.

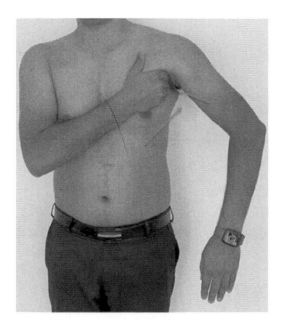

Step 2: Grab one side of your chest and move it upward towards the armpit. Do this ten times.

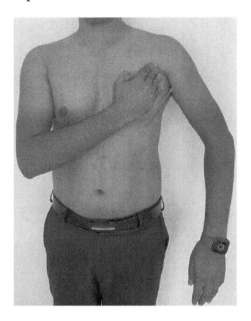

Step 3: Holding your chest stable, pump the upper inner quadrant of one side up towards your neck. Do this five times.

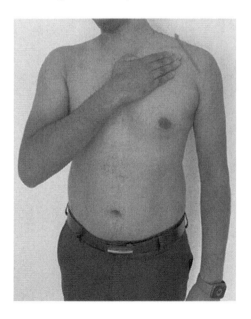

Step 4: You can do the pumping more than the recommended number of times if you like.

Step 5: Massage the operated area in circular motions using any moisturising lotion or massage oil with your hands. The massage should be done twice a day for 20 to30 minutes. Moderate pressure should be used when massaging. For the first week, the pressure on the stitches needs to be light. Following the first week, the pressure can be equally moderate in all the areas. While massaging, the patient may sometimes notice areas of hardness or even have areas that seem filled with liquid. Unless it is extensive, it will reduce gradually with the massage.

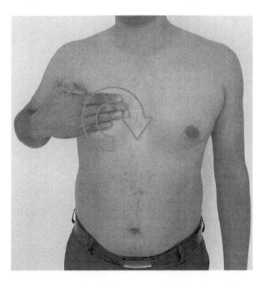

Some patients hire a massage therapist two to three times per week, but that may be unnecessary. Massage is best done before a shower as the patient will be able to wash off the lotion/oil and lessen the chances of blocking skin pores.

There are other adjuvants therapies to reduce swelling faster. These include multipolar cavitation radio frequency, vacuum therapy, etc. These are sometimes used in patients in whom the swelling is refractory and takes longer than usual to reduce. Some surgeons even offer these sessions as a part of the surgical package. Any of these therapies would involve multiple sessions of what feels like a mechanised massage. The results are usually visible in four to six sessions. While this is by no means mandatory, they are definitely useful in selected cases.

Incisions and Healing: After the surgery, the patient is seen back in the clinic to have the contoured areas inspected. Absorbable sutures are not removed and they usually dissolve and fall off in 10-20 days. Avoiding direct sunlight to the incision line is advisable as this may result in pigmentation changes. This is particularly true during the first year after the surgery. It's better not to expose the incision to sunlight without sunblock—of SPF 30 or greater. Scars will initially be red and a little raised but, over three to six months, they usually get lighter in colour and flatten out.

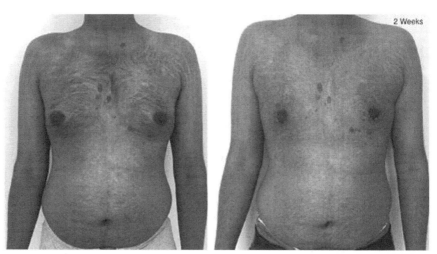

Before and two weeks after surgery. Notice the absorbable white sutures still in place in the picture on the right

In some unfortunate individuals, there is an excess scarring tendency that may lead to hypertrophic scarring or keloids. These are extensions of unchecked scar formation and is difficult to predict and more difficult to treat. These scars look raised, harder and larger than regular scars and lead to significant cosmetic blemish and psychological distress. Some men who may be susceptible to such scarring tend to face such issues. If the patient has abnormal scarring in any other part of the body, it is advisable to bring it to the notice of the surgeon before the surgery so that he can take steps and precautions to lessen the chances of such scarring after gynecomastia surgery. The precautions include anti-scar creams, silicone gel and sheets, mild steroid injections, pressure therapy, etc. Silicone gels and sheets are adhesive, soft and semi-occlusive dressing that have been a popular topical treatment for various scars and is supported by many systematic reviews of the evidence for its effectiveness. However, there is no fool-proof method to entirely avoid hypertrophic scars and keloids in a predisposed individual with any method. Once the excess scars do form after the surgery, the treatment usually starts with steroid (commonly Triamcinolone) injection into the scars. These will make the scars more supple, flatter and less itchy. Multiple sessions of such injections may be needed.

Bruises are a common occurrence after any liposuction and gynecomastia is no different. The fairer the individual, the more is he predisposed to bruising. It is noticeable usually from the second day of surgery. It is maroon or blue in colour and gradually fades after it turns brown. Massage and compression vests help the bruises heal faster. Some creams may also be advised in excess bruising.

Your Daily Operated Site Care Schedule-To be followed in the Morning and Evening

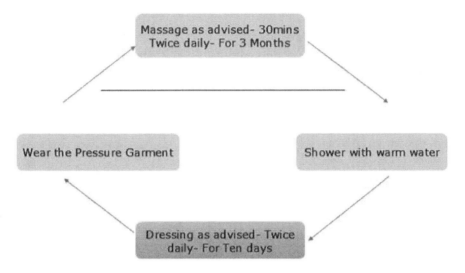

Posture after Surgery: As discussed earlier, it's common to see people with gynecomastia hunch forward while walking. This is a bad physical trait that leads to postural and spinal issues in the future. During the follow-up, it is paramount that the surgeon stresses the importance of consciously avoiding that. The patients should be aware that the breasts are gone and they don't have to hunch anymore to hide it. They need to walk straight with their chin up. Occasionally, a visit to the physiotherapist or chiropractor is beneficial. Also, men tend to return to wearing proper fitting shirts as opposed to the loose shirts they are used to wearing.

Chapter 7

COMPLICATIONS OF GYNECOMASTIA SURGERY

Gynecomastia though is a common surgery for which complications are, thankfully, very rare. Let's discuss them in detail:

1. **Collection:** A gynecomastia surgery creates a potential space under the skin where the gland once was. This space, until it collapses can accumulate blood (Hematoma) or clear body fluids (Seroma) or a combination of both (Hemato-Seroma). Theoretically, it occurs in about three to five percent of the cases. This may be noticed once the surgical dressing is removed after two to three days. The patient feels like there is fluid in the operated areas and, if the collection is large enough, it may cause a significant swelling of the chest, even mimicking the patient's original breasts. This needs a visit to the doctor to get it checked. While collection itself is not serious in most cases, the healing and results may get delayed due to this.

   Once the surgeon checks the collection, he may feel the need to take it out (aspirate). This may be done with a syringe or a small opening may be done in the incision so as to evacuate the collection. The decision of evacuating the collection may be deferred depending on the amount and nature of the collection. If the surgeon feels that the collection is small enough for the body to absorb it in a few days, then no aspiration is needed and the patient may continue with compression garments and massages.

Even if the amount of collection is large, the surgeon may sometimes defer aspiration to allow for the collection to get liquefied. In many cases, trying to aspirate too early is futile as the collection is in a semi-solid, jelly-like state. This decision is taken clinically by the surgeon upon examination. Once the aspiration is done, the compression garments are a must to avoid re-accumulation.

2. **Delayed Wound Healing:** Once the stitches are put over the incision, it is expected to heal uneventfully in about seven to ten days. However, in a few individuals, the healing may get delayed due to various factors like:

- Excessive smoking
- Diabetes
- Other health issues that may affect healing
- Use of steroids
- Excessive and early motion of the operated site
- Lifting of weights too early
- Excessive collection at the operated site
- Excessive tension on the operated site, especially if loose skin was removed during the surgery
- Infection

In a smoker, it is always advisable to defect the surgery for at least three weeks so that he can reduce smoking as much as he realistically can. This is neither a rule nor a guarantee that wound healing will be optimal after three weeks. It, however, betters the chances for an optimal healing. This is applicable in chain-smokers and even drug abusers.

Diabetes is not a contraindication for the surgery and the only requirement is that the sugars be controlled before, during and after the surgery. During the pre-operative tests, if the sugars are unreasonably high, they should be controlled before the surgery can be scheduled. During the surgery, the anaesthetist monitors the sugars and, after the surgery, more advice is given so as to keep the sugars in check.

There are other health issues that may adversely impact healing. These include Bronchial Asthma, steroid use or abuse for any reason, cardiac health issues and many other reasons for which the list can be endless. The presence of such issues is not only rare in the usual gynecomastia population, but they are also screened for clinically by the surgeon. Presence of any such health issues can be clinically detected by the patient's history and during the clinical examination. If there is a clue to the presence of any such issues, the surgeon may advise more tests or even refer him to the concerned physician before the surgery can be undertaken. Such consultations may occasionally become necessary if the healing is unduly prolonged.

Once the surgery is done and the stitches are put, the operated area should not move vigorously. This is the reason why a large dressing with multiple layers is put onto the operated area. Too early and too vigorous movements of the chest may put excessive strain on the stitches and may even lead them to open up. Once that happens, the optimal healing cycle breaks and starts all over again, thus delaying healing.

3. **Infection:** A clean surgery like gynecomastia is unlikely to get infected. There are occasional circumstances where an infection does occur at the operated site. Infection is also among the rarer causes of delayed wound healing. The signs of infection include:

   • Redness over the chest that's a little different from post-procedure bruising

   • Excess itching and pain

   • Fever

   • Chills

- Excess sweating
- Pus discharge form the incision
- Delayed healing
- A swelling that's tender, painful and does not resolve in time

The CDC (Centres for Disease Control and prevention) describes three types of surgical site infections (SSI):

1. Superficial incisional SSI – This infection occurs just in the area of the skin where the incision was made.

2. Deep incisional SSI – This infection occurs beneath the incision area in muscle and the tissues surrounding the muscles.

3. Organ or space SSI – This type of infection can be in any area of the body other than skin, muscle and surrounding tissue that was involved in the surgery. This includes a body organ or a space between organs.

Any SSI may cause redness, delayed healing, fever, pain, tenderness, warmth or swelling. These are the other signs and symptoms for specific types of SSI:

- A superficial incisional SSI may produce pus from the wound site. Samples of the pus may be grown in a culture to find out the types of germs that are causing the infection.

- A deep incisional SSI may also produce pus. The wound site may reopen on its own or a surgeon may reopen the wound and find pus inside the wound.

- An organ or space SSI may show a discharge of pus coming from a drain placed through the skin into a body space or organ. A collection of pus, called an abscess, is an enclosed area of pus and disintegrating tissue surrounded by inflammation. An abscess may be seen when the surgeon reopens the wound or by special X-ray studies.

These infections occur in men with predisposing factors like

- Very young or very old age
- Poorly controlled diabetes
- Smokers
- Steroid use
- Compromised immune system
- Infection or colonisation at a remote body site
- Obesity
- Poor nutritional status
- Length of pre-operative stay (increases exposure to pathogens)
- Wound contamination

These features, as described by the Hopkin's Institute and CDC, though generally to all surgeries, apply aptly to gynecomastia surgery too. Once the features of infection are noted, a review by the surgeon is mandatory. The surgeon would then, depending on the extent of infection, advise antibiotics, culture of pus or, sometimes, drainage of the pus. The drainage of pus is usually done through the original incision or via another incision depending on the site and extent of infection. The infection needs to be controlled and treated in time for the eventual desired cosmetic results.

4. **Unfavourable scarring:** The scar is of a major concern in gynecomastia patients. I have seen many being disproportionately concerned the scarring and having deferred the surgery for a long time. Of the many incisions described for gynecomastia surgery, most leave a scar that is not very obvious. However, the peril-areolar or intra-areolar incision leaves the most subtle scars. The reason for the peril-areolar scar being well-hidden is because it lies at the junction of the darker and pigmented areola and the surrounding, normal skin. Hence, once the healing is complete,

the scars look like a transition area between the dark and the fairer skin around the areola. The intra-areolar sera is also quite well-hidden in the small skin folds of the areola. However, it may sometimes leave a visible scar if the scar becomes even minimally hypo-pigmented. This means, sometimes, scars loose pigment (colour) that is usually temporary. This shows up due to its contrast from the surrounding darker skin while such loss of pigment may not be an issue in the peri-areolar scars.

Apart from the normally healed scars, sometimes, excess scarring may result in keloids or hypertrophic scars. Once they do occur in the unfortunate predisposed individuals, there needs to be regular follow-up with the surgeon to work out the best treatment options.

5. **Breast Asymmetry and contour irregularities:** It is a common finding to see asymmetric breasts among Gynecomastia patients. However, one of the targets of a gynecomastia surgery is to achieve symmetry as much as possible. This is far easier in men who have a symmetric breast to begin with. Asymmetry can result from various reasons:

- Excess or less liposuction on one side
- Excess or less removal of the gland
- A combination of the two
- A pre-existing asymmetry
- Asymmetric skin folds and looseness

Every effort is done to avoid such scenarios after the surgery. Once they do occur, the treatment is tricky and depends on the amount and location of asymmetry. The options now would include a couple of revision surgeries, selective liposuction or even fat grafting. One of the advantages of the superior dynamic flap method is this very situation. By this method, the chances of such issues are rare as the tissue can be mobilised to the area the surgeon desires. Moreover, even doing the revision surgeries to correct any asymmetries, since the blood supply of the remaining breast tissue is intact, it can again be placed in the area where it is required to correct the asymmetry.

Contour irregularities are shape irregularities. They can be in the form of visible bumps or depression or the dreaded 'crater deformity.' Most of the irregularities may be minor enough for both the surgeon and the patient to overlook. Sometimes though, the irregularities need to be treated for the desired result. The treatment depends on the nature, content and extent of the irregularity or asymmetry.

In cases where there is a noticeable bulge due to fat, a simple liposuction under local anaesthesia will suffice. If the bulge is due to gland remnants, then an open excision may be needed wherein the surgeon will most likely make a cut through the old scar and remove the culprit glandular tissue.

If the issue is a depression, then the treatment is slightly trickier. If the depression is in an area where the remaining gland can be mobilised without affecting its primary function (the purpose of the gland remnant is to contour the chest aesthetically after the procedure), then the gland can be re-mobilised to augment the depressed area. This will involve a re-surgery which most likely will involve opening through the old scars. In most cases, such revisions can be done under local anaesthesia. If the depression is in an area where the gland cannot be mobilised, or if it is large enough, then various options would be considered. The most common among them is fat grafting.

Fat grafting is a procedure wherein fat is harvested by doing a small liposuction at another part of the body (like abdomen or thigh) and then purified (centrifuged) and injected into the depressed areas to correct the contour irregularities. Fat grafting has been in use for various applications in plastic surgery like breast augmentation, buttock augmentation, augmentation of facial structures and correcting deformities among others. It works predictably and perfectly in areas that are not scarred. But, in scarred areas—like after a gynecomastia surgery—it is slightly more unpredictable. This is to do with how transferred fat survives. When fat is transferred from one area to another, it gets its blood supply from the surrounding tissues. In scarred areas, this blood supply may be impeded due to the surgical trauma and injury. This makes fat grafting a little less predictable. However, fat grafting does achieve good contour correction especially if done over multiple sessions for scarred areas. Though this may be cumbersome for the patient, the chances of the transferred fat surviving predictably are higher.

It is not unusual to see a combination of visible bumps and depressions over the chest following surgery. In a few cases, the patients are stressed about these issues more than they did for the gynecomastia to begin with and rightfully so. When bumps occur in combination with depressed areas, the surgeon will have to assess all the operated areas to obtain clues about the causes. The treatment in such cases is usually a combination of liposuction, gland excision, gland mobilisation and fat grafting. The best way to treat such issues is to avoid them.

6. **Chest skin swelling, bruising and ecchymosis:** Bruising and swelling occur in almost all liposuction patients immediately after the procedure. It is considered more of a sequel as a part of recovery than a complication. It reaches its peak by seven to ten days and then generally disappears by two to four weeks after the surgery. The extent of bruising again depends on the nature and colour of skin. It is severe in fair+ skin and the least in darker skin. Excessive bruising/ecchymosis is related

to smoking, use of medications for thinning blood and other bleeding/clotting disorders. Very rarely, it may be related to bleeding from superficial veins damaged during the liposuction procedure.

To reduce the extent of bruising, smokers are advised to stop smoking for at least three weeks prior to major liposuction and blood thinners are stopped with a physician's clearance at least a week prior to surgery. It is also advisable to check the patient's bleeding and clotting profile prior to the surgery.

Once the bruising sets in, it gradually reduces over a few weeks and during this time, the colour changes from maroon, blue, brown and then pale brown. Massage and pressure garments help reduce the bruising faster.

7. **Change in skin sensation:** Following gynecomastia it is not rare to see a few patients feel reduced or altered sensation over the chest. This tends to last for up to six months after the surgery. This is due to damage to the microscopic covering of small nerves that provide sensation to the chest skin. This, however, is rarely a persistent issue and settles down on its own in time.

Very rarely, some men develop neuromas that tend to be painful and persist for a long time. Such patients need to visit the surgeon again, who may advise aesthetic injection or rarely a small surgery to treat the neuroma, leading to depolarisation of the cutaneous sensory nerves.

Hypoaesthesia is very common after liposuction but sensations generally return to near normal by the end of one year. Chronic pain is rare and may be due to a neuroma or due to injury to underlying fascia or muscle. Multiple injections of local anaesthetic may be helpful. Unrelenting pain may require surgical release of scar with or without AFT.

Long-standing hyperaesthesia has been reported following UAL. This is due to damage to the phospholipids in the myelin sheath leading to depolarisation of the cutaneous sensory nerves.

8. **Looseness of skin:** Looseness or laxity of chest skin after gynecomastia is one of the underestimated post-procedure issues. There are a few reasons why someone's skin does not reshape well after the procedure. It is more common in higher grades of gynecomastia, older age, larger glands. smokers, diabetics, people who have a lot of weight fluctuations, etc.

This should, however, not be a major issue in grades I and IIA especially if they belong to skin tone grading T. Very rarely, there may be minimal looseness in those with poor skin tone (Grade L). In higher grades there are chances of loose skin after gynecomastia surgery. In my practice, I have noticed such issues in about five to ten percent of men with grade IIB and a much higher percentage in grade III although I guess it should be around 30 to 40 percent. Of course, those who start with the L grading tend to fare worse.

The extent of laxity also depends on the nature of skin. Dermatologically, the skin is classified into six categories. This is famously referred to as Fitzpatrick classification. Though this primarily highlights the colour and the response of skin to sunlight, it also indicates the nature of overall skin tone. Though not scientifically proven, I have noticed that the higher the number, typer-wise as per the classification, the better the skin tends to retract after surgery. Most Indians fall under type IV or V. Indian skin tone is generally better than western skin and the skin too shrinks a little better and more predictably. This is probably one of the reasons why post-gynecomastia skin looseness is much more common in fairer western skin than most Indians.

Fitzpatrick Classification of Skin Types I through VI

Type I	Type II	Type III	Type IV	Type V	Type VI
White skin. Always burns, never tans.	Fair skin. Always burns, tans with difficulty.	Average skin colour. Sometimes mild burn, tan about average.	Light-brown skin. Rarely burns. Tans easily.	Brown skin. Never burns. Tans very easily.	Black skin. Heavily pigmented. Never burns, tans very easily.

Here are some methods to reduce the chances of loose skin after gynecomastia surgery:

1. Start massaging the chest as soon as your surgeon clears you.
2. Continue massage as long as possible, longer for higher grades.
3. Avoid smoking.
4. Correct blood sugars of you are a diabetic.
5. Start chest workouts gradually after about three weeks. The constant stretching and muscle movements tend to make the skin shrink better.
6. Wear the pressure garment diligently as advised by the surgeon.
7. Make sure the garment is tight and stays tight. Get it re-tightened if necessary.

However, once the looseness sets it, managing it is a difficult task. There are various surgical and non-surgical options to manage the loose skin. It also depends on the amount of looseness. Before deciding on opting for treatment for the looseness, it is advisable to try workouts, massages and garments for a longer duration. The treatment options will be assessed by the surgeon once the individual exhausts the above options. Therapies include radio frequency skin tightening, lasers, ultrasound or, as a final option, surgical skin tightening.

Surgical skin tightening may be a necessity in higher grades with a lot of loose skin to begin with. Many surgeons plan the skin tightening at a later date, a few months down the line after the primary gynecomastia surgery. The rationale is that, as the individual wears the garment and works out, the skin will tighten up to a considerable extent. This, in turn, reduces the scarring of the eventual skin tightening surgery. Some surgeons, however, do skin tightening at the time of the first surgery. I fall into the first group. I prefer to wait and reduce the scarring as much as possible. This is especially true in Indian skin where the scars may not be as aesthetic as in fairer skin.

9. **Skin Necrosis:** Like any other part of the body, the skin too needs a certain amount of blood supply to heal when injured or cut. So, when an incision is made during gynecomastia surgery, this blood supply is temporarily cut. But, because the incision is small and the blood vessels supplying the skin travel very close to the skin surface, the healing is very rarely compromised. However, in some instances, the healing may get delayed due to inadequate blood supply or, sometimes, some parts of the skin may necrose or die. Though thankfully this is very rare, there are a few factors which may increase the chances of skin necrosis:

   • Too aggressive dissection during the surgery.

   • Dissection very close to the skin surface that may damage the blood supply to the areola and nipple.

   • Patient factors like uncontrolled diabetes, excessive smoking or connective tissue disorders that may have reduced the blood supply in the first place.

- Post-procedure complication like large collection that may hamper blood supply.
- Repeated surgeries.

In most cases, this skin necrosis is limited to a small area in the incision. This is usually limited to an areas healing later than the surrounding parts of the incision. Usually, this tends to be area where the liposuction was done from-usually the centre most points. This is also because it is the farthest from intact blood supply. These are easily treated by just taking care of the wounds till they heal. Occasionally though, they made need scar revisions, as such delayed healing leaves wider scars.

In very rare instances, a large part of the areola and nipple may necrose. This starts with very delayed healing, followed by some part of the areola turning black and, later, this skin peels, leaving behind scars which may be discoloured. The issue here is a discoloured nipple and areola which end up not being very aesthetic. Once this does happen, the surgeon may advise a minor surgery to correct it. There are different methods to correct it including skin grafts, false surgeries and nipple grafts act. Most of these procedures are minor and can be done under local anaesthesia and yield acceptable results once the healing is complete.

10. **Reaction to dressing materials, tapes or ointments:** A few men can be allergic to the materials used for the stitches or even the dressing materials. They present with reddish appearance of skin accompanied by pain and itching. When identified early, it can be easily treated by stopping the offending agent and switching to a substitute. Occasionally, a dermatologist's opinion may be need in severe cases.

In a scenario called suture sinus, the patient may notice a small opening with occasional pus or watery discharge. It is due to the allergy to the material the stitches are made of. It is treated with local antiseptic creams, antibiotics or a minor procedure called incision and drainage, if needed.

11. **Damage to deeper structures:** A few patients do ask me whether the heart can get injured during liposuction. Any plastic surgeon is usually trained enough to make sure the instruments stay in the areas where the fat and glands are present. So the chances of injuring deeper structures like the heart and lungs are almost unheard of. However, the underlying muscle, the pectoralis major, may get injured during rough liposuction. In most cases, it presents a persistent and severe pain and stiffness. It usually heals without any intervention except rest and timed physiotherapy. Some minor nerves do get damaged during the procedures and may lead to loss or reduction of sensation over the chest area. However, this is usually temporary and it settles down in a few months.

12. **Fat embolism:** Fat embolism is a phenomenon where small globules of fat escape into major blood vessels and may lead to lung or heart dysfunction. Fat embolism syndrome is a commonly documented complication of traumatic injuries (one to five percent after long-bone fracture), but it is very rare after liposuction. Only a few cases have been reported. It is so rare that it is often under-diagnosed especially as many recover without sever symptoms. Due to the low specificity and sensitivity of laboratory tests and physical examination and the diagnostic confusion with other syndromes (for example, thromboembolism, myocardial infarction, acute respiratory distress syndrome, among others), there is often a delay in the diagnosis. The classic triad involving acute respiratory failure, neurological dysfunction and petechiae is very rarely seen. The patients who do suffer from this present with severe breathing difficulty, chest pain, fainting episodes, etc. Some tests that are advised include serum lipase, tests of lipids in urine and MRI scans. The treatment is supportive and

includes the management of the airway and lung dysfunction, hemodynamic, and steroids.

13. **Deep vein thrombosis, heart and lung complications:** Deep vein thrombosis (DVT) is when a blood clot in the leg. This clot can sometimes travel to lung (Pulmonary thromboembolism, PE) or heart and causes severe issues and even death. These issues are the most common causes of death after liposuction. However, this is thankfully rare. The chances of this are higher after prolonged immobilisation or clotting abnormalities in the individual. If a patient presents with severe chest pain and breathlessness, PE is one of the diagnosis to be borne in mind. Such patients need to be treated in an ICU. Treatment includes pharmacologic therapy with thrombolytics (that will dissolve clots) and anticoagulation (to prevent further clotting) and supportive treatment.

14. **Anaesthesia risks:** The chances of anaesthetic complications depend on the setup where it is performed, amount of fat removed, surgical time taken, patients existing health issues, etc. The causes of death reported following liposuction have been—cardiac arrest due to fluid overload, pulmonary oedema, lignocaine toxicity, fat embolism and acute respiratory distress syndrome (ARDS). Such complications can be readily avoided by:

- Adequate pre-surgical screening by the surgeon and anaesthetist.
- Proper pre-surgical work-up and tests.
- Surgery in a healthy individual.
- Surgery done in a fully equipped centre.
- Experienced surgeon and anaesthetist.

Anaesthesia for gynecomastia surgery requires a thorough understanding of the physiological changes and likely complications associated with them. Meticulous planning, monitoring and strict adherence to guidelines for fluid therapy ensures a good outcome. In many cases, patients are advised to meet the anaesthetist beforehand (Pre-Anaesthetic Evaluation, PAE), especially if he has any health issues to begin with or if his tests show up something unexpected.

TOP SURGERY FOR TRANS MEN

Trans men are those who have been attributed to female sex at birth. But, when they mature, they self-identify as men. Many trans men look for male breast surgery or, as commonly called, Top Surgery. With this, they attempt to reduce their feminine chest shape.

Although breast/chest appearance is an important secondary sex characteristic, breast presence or size is not involved in the legal definitions of sex and gender and is not necessary for reproduction. The performance of breast/chest operations for the treatment of gender dysphoria should be considered with the same care as beginning hormone therapy as both produce relatively irreversible changes to the body.

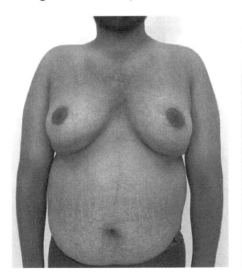 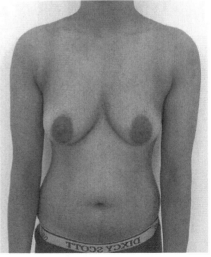

The greats in Trans men resembles a grade III Gynecomastia

This Top surgery is done in individuals who have begun taking testosterone and after they have been adjusting themselves socially as males. The World Professional Association for Transgender Health (WPATH) lays down standards of care that require:

1. Letter assuring consent for surgery from a psychiatrist/mental health provider.

2. Though most individuals undergoing top surgery are 18 or older, younger individuals may be considered for the procedure if the patient, their legal guardians and their mental health professional are in agreement that top surgery is appropriate.

3. The best candidates for top surgery are those who are mature enough to fully understand the procedure and have realistic expectations about the results.

4. Male chest reconstruction is not recommended for trans-masculine persons who intend to breast-feed.

5. There is persistent, well-documented gender dysphoria.

6. Capacity to make a fully informed decision and to consent for treatment.

7. Age of the majority in a given country.

8. If significant medical or mental health concerns are present, they must be reasonably well controlled.

The approach to trans persons seeking for a mastectomy is illustrated by the Standards of Care of the World Professional Association of Transgender Health.

Many protocols to choose the most appropriate surgical technique are based on anatomical parameters. Generally, the smaller the breast the smaller the incisions required; on the other hand, the larger or more loose the breast tissue, the larger the incisions required.

The social stigma attached to such issues is very well researched. These individuals are strongly advised to seek regular counselling.

Strong family support and social life are vital for a better outlook.

Doctors who perform surgical treatments for breasts in gender dysphoria should be plastic surgeons who are board-certified as such by the relevant national councils. In many cases, these can be treated like any other gynecomastia. However, in some cases, they may need a skin tightening surgery at a later date to fully achieve an aesthetic chest.

Chapter 8

RESULTS AFTER SURGERY

It is widely considered that plastic surgery is a balanced combination of science and art. But, when dealing with patients especially in gynecomastia, this art needs a scientific background and assessment. Since beauty is subjective, so too are the results of aesthetic results of a gynecomastia surgery. Many men with breasts get surgeries done for a combination of physical and psychological reasons. Like any aesthetic surgery, it is imperative for both the surgeons and the patients to be able to assess their results in such a way that they can be both objective and easy to assess and follow-up. While assessment questionnaires are available and are quite widely used, it is usually the patient and the surgeon who are best placed to assess the results. As with most aesthetic surgeries, a photographic documentation of the individual's progress is vital for sharing information of the progress of the individual and for a more effective audit of the surgeon's technique. After the surgery, the relief is quite dramatic in larger glands, both aesthetically and psychologically and hence the satisfaction and aesthetic improvements are also significantly higher. Here are some results of various grades and types for reference:

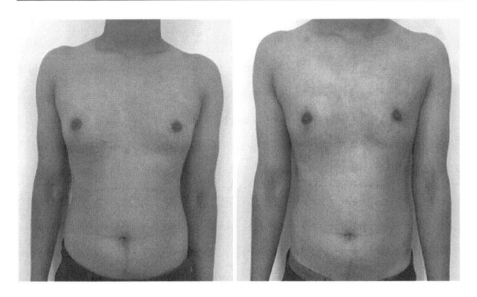

18-year-old with Grade I Gynecomastia

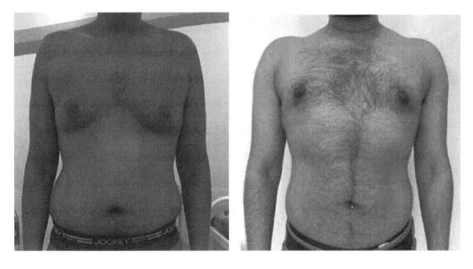

46-year-old with Grade IIB Gynecomastia-Also underwent abdomen
Liposuction

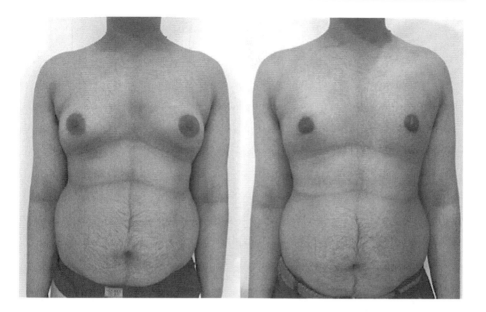

28-year-old with Grade IIB Gynecomastia

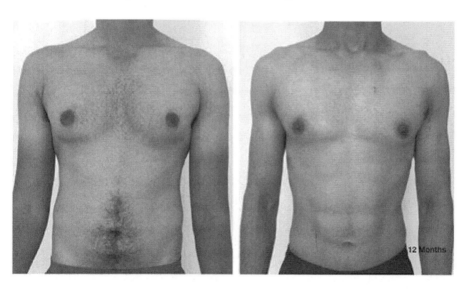

32-year-old with Grade IIA Gynecomastia

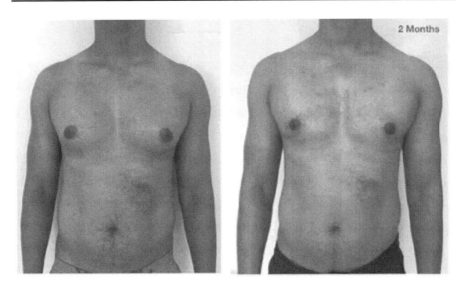

29-year-old with Grade IIA Gynecomastia—also underwent abdomen Liposuction

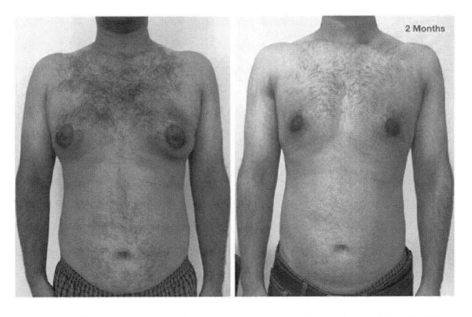

32-year-old with Grade IIA Gynecomastia on the right and Grade IIB Gynecomastia on left

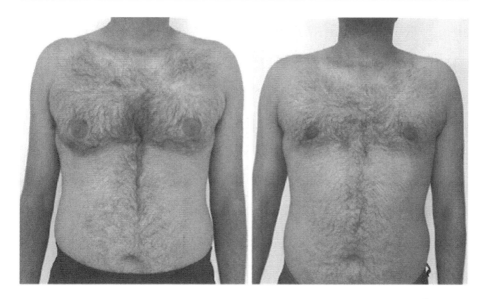

37-year-old with Grade IIA Gynecomastia

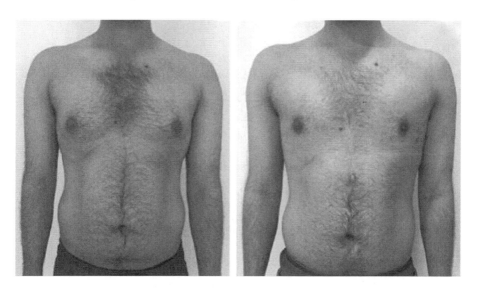

19-year-old with Grade IIB Gynecomastia

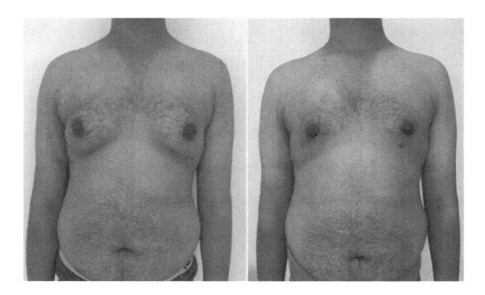

23-year-old with Grade IIA Gynecomastia

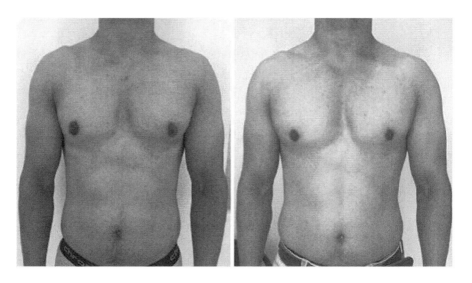

A 29-year-old bodybuilder with Grade IIA Gynecomastia

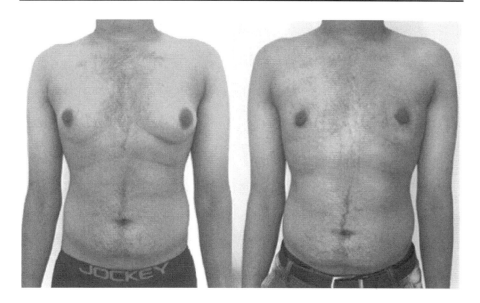

31-year-old with Grade IIA Gynecomastia

RE-OCCURRENCE AFTER GYNECOMASTIA SURGERY

Many patients ask me this question. As a rule of thumb, breast tissue cannot grow back after puberty. But, like any rule, this one too has exceptions. Though gynecomastia is idiopathic in many cases, the rare Secondary Gynecomastia may predispose the patient for re-occurrence. This is especially true in drug addicts, marijuana smokers etc. When such causes are not corrected, there is a theoretical chance that the breast tissue may enlarge or even regrow. However, in my practice I have hardly notice such reoccurrences.

Another scenario is where such breast can be regarded is in the hormone producing tumour in the body. When such active tumours produce excess quantities of gynecomastia inducing hormones, there is a chance the gynecomastia can reoccur. Here, the gynecomastia results from an imbalance between estradiol and testosterone and, in such scenarios, comprehensive hormone analysis and other tests to detect the culprit tutor may be needed. Rarely, this can also occur due to steroid abuse and due to the side effects of certain medications.

The most common scenario, where someone says that his gynecomastia has come back, is in people who put on a lot of weight after surgery. When fat cells are removed during liposuction, they cannot grow back. But if the patient's diet, exercise and lifestyle patterns are unhealthy, the remixing fat cells can get bigger and mimic gynecomastia. This excess fat, accompanied by the internal scarring from the previous surgery, closely mimics gynecomastia. The surgeon may sometimes find it hard to differentiate. However, in such cases it is better to alter the lifestyle than directly going under the knife again.

Another scenario where the patient feels his breast has grown back is when inadequate removal of the breast was done in the first place. In such individuals, a re-surgery is needed.

Chapter 9

CONCLUSION

For an issue that nearly affects 60 percent of men, it is indeed surprising that there is so little genuine information available out there. While the internet is flooded with anecdotes and misinformation, there is no way for a common man to assess the authenticity of such information. As someone who deals with gynecomastia patients every day, I felt it was my responsibility to cover all facets of gynecomastia and provide as objective an opinion as possible.

Anyway, there are some things that I would like to stress here. The mental aspect of someone with a male breast should not be underestimated. If your child or a friend shows signs that these may be related, the least you can do is to ask him to meet an expert in treating it. Neglecting it may only worsen the said issues. Though there are many medical treatments that have been tried for gynecomastia, success has been precious little. Surgery remains the gold standard in treating gynecomastia. A combination of liposuction and excision of the gland is an ideal combination barring few exceptions.

Chapter 10

GYNECOMASTIA SURGERY QANDA

1. What is gynecomastia?

Gynecomastia is a medical term that comes from the Greek words for "women-like breasts." Gynecomastia affects an estimated 40 to 60 percent of Indian men. For men who feel self-conscious about their appearance, male breast reduction surgery can help. The surgery removes fat and/or glandular tissue from the breasts and, in extreme cases, removes excess skin, resulting in a chest that is flatter, firmer and better contoured.

2. Am I a good candidate for male breast reduction surgery?

Before considering surgery, the most important question you should ask yourself is: does the condition bother you psychologically, socially and/or physically? If the answer is yes, you should consider surgery and start to gather the information that will help you make an intelligent decision while consulting a plastic surgeon experienced in this type of surgery.

WHO IS A GOOD CANDIDATE FOR GYNECOMASTIA SURGERY?

MEN WITH REALISTIC EXPECTATIONS

MEN WITHOUT A MEDICAL CONDITION OR LIFE-THREATENING ILLNESSES THAT CAN DELAY HEALING

NONSMOKERS AND NON-DRUG USERS

MEN WITH A POSITIVE OUTLOOK

MEN WHO ARE PHYSICALLY HEALTHY

MEN WHO ARE BOTHERED BY THEIR BREASTS

www.gynecomastiabangalore.com

Here is a list of pointers that make one a good candidate to undergo gynecomastia surgery:

- Men without major skin disorders involving the chest area.

- Men who are bothered by the feeling that their breasts are too large.

- Men whose breast development has stabilised.

- Men who are physically healthy and have a stable weight.

- Men with specific goals in mind for improving the symptoms of gynecomastia.

- Men with a positive outlook.

- Non-smokers and non-drug users.

- Men who do not have a medical condition or life-threatening illnesses that can delay healing.

- Men with realistic expectations.

3. Can gynecomastia be treated with diet and exercise?

Diet and exercise are to be strongly recommended—they are great for your general health. However, it is a common misconception that diligent and long-term exercises reduce or even eliminate male breasts. It is routine to see an individual presenting to us with gynecomastia saying that he had worked as hard as he could, but he could not "burn the breast." The main problem is in the understanding of male breasts—gynecomastia.

Exercise does not burn the breast tissue. The common misconception is that the breast tissue is made of fat. It is made of the *Breast Gland*. Hence it can't be burnt, no matter the amount of exercise or workouts. What exercise does, however, is, it enlarges the chest muscle called the pectoralis major which lies beneath the breast tissue. So, when the muscle increases in size and bulk, it only makes the breast tissue look more prominent and hence worsens the overall appearance. Adding to this, people take protein supplements that may have small amounts of anabolic steroids or hormones. It further increases the muscle bulk and also increases the prominence of breast tissues.

4. What is the ideal age to undergo gynecomastia surgery?

Traditionally, it was viewed that one should undergo gynecomastia surgery only after puberty and around 16 to 18 years. Unfortunately, many teenagers spend their entire teenage years waiting for the surgery and are subject to ridicule and embarrassment during this critical time in their lives. Many people even think that gynecomastia resolves on its own after puberty, which is a very rare occurrence. It is important to notice the state of the breast gland for up to two years. If it has increased, or is the same, then it is prudent to plan the procedure. The decision to operate is based not only on the diagnosis of gynecomastia but also on the physical and mental maturity of the person and his capability of understanding the surgery as well as the ability to cope with the post-operative pain and follow the post-operative care regimen. Surgery has been successfully performed on hundreds of young men from ages 12 through 18. This decision is made is on an individual basis.

Men older than 45 years suffering from gynecomastia are also candidates for surgery, but must understand that the skin may not fully tighten after the surgery is performed since they may have lost some elasticity in their skin through the natural process of ageing.

5. How is the gynecomastia graded?

The extent and severity of gynecomastia are graded by many methods. The commonly used method is Clark's classification. It grades the gynecomastia based on the amount of breast tissue and the extent of loose skin over the breast. Clinically, gynecomastia is graded as follows:

Grade 1: Small enlargement, but without excess skin over the chest

Grade 2a: Moderate enlargement, without excess skin over the chest

Grade 2b: Moderate enlargement with extra skin over the chest

Grade 3: Marked enlargement with extra skin over the chest.

6. How do I know which grade I belong to?

The grade of gynecomastia of a person is best assessed by a plastic surgeon as he can assess the amount of tissue and laxity of skin better.

7. Is there a risk of cancer if I have gynecomastia?

Gynecomastia does not make one more prone to breast cancer. Many studies have concluded that there is no increased risk of male breast cancer in men with gynecomastia. It is important to note, however, that one percent of all breast cancers do occur in men. While it is very rarely seen in young men, older men must be made aware of this possibility. Therefore, any new lump, one-sided growth (asymmetry of the breast), skin changes of the breast or nipple, or bloody nipple discharge should be immediately investigated by a doctor. Cancer usually occurs in older men. A biopsy, a mammogram or a sonogram (ultrasound) examination may be advised. If in doubt, it is best to get it checked by a surgeon.

8. Will the treatment vary if I have asymmetric breasts?

It is very common to have asymmetric breasts in all grades of gynecomastia. Unilateral (one-sided) gynecomastia is also a fairly common occurrence. On such occasions, the surgeon will assess the need for surgery, mode of surgery and surgical type based on the individual case. Careful examination of both breasts is performed and surgery on both breasts is considered if need be. If this smaller amount of gynecomastia is not addressed at surgery, then the result may be that the operated side will look completely normal and the un-operated side may not look bulky. It is extremely difficult to operate on the larger side and reduce it just enough to match the other side. Thus, appropriate surgery should be done to optimise both sides at the same time. The other issue with one-sided gynecomastia is to be very sure that it is not a tumour and hence should be checked on a priority basis.

9. What are the causes of gynecomastia?

The cause of gynecomastia is a widely researched topic. Many studies reveal multiple causes and multiple classifications. For understanding, it is easier to classify the causes as primary or secondary. Primary (also called idiopathic or unknown) gynecomastia is one where the cause is unknown, though various genetic factors are associated with it. Secondary Gynecomastia is where the cause is identifiable like hormonal issues, tumours, drug overuse or abuse.

Some estimates suggest the following causes in males seeking medical attention for gynecomastia:

- Persistent Pubertal (teenage) Gynecomastia—25 percent
- No detectable abnormality—25 percent
- Drugs—10-25 percent
- Liver disorders or malnutrition—8 percent
- Primary hypogonadism (Underdeveloped testes)—8 percent
- Testicular tumours—3 percent
- Secondary hypogonadism—2 percent
- Hyperthyroidism—1.5 percent
- Chronic renal insufficiency—1 percent

These statistics are primarily of the western population. In India, Primary Gynecomastia is far more common and probably accounts for 90 percent of cases. Secondary causes account for the rest. It is, however, important to clinically assess the probable causes and then advise tests only if necessary.

10. What is assessed during the first consultation?

At first consultation, all patients require a thorough history and physical exam. Particular attention should be given to medications, drug and alcohol abuse as well as other chemical exposures. Symptoms of underlying systemic illness, such as hyperthyroidism, liver disease or renal failure should be sought. Furthermore, the clinician will assess tumours as a possible cause and should establish the duration and timing of breast development. Rapid and/or painful breast growth that has occurred recently is more concerning than a long-standing gynecomastia. Additionally, the clinician should inquire about fertility, erectile dysfunction and libido to rule out hypogonadism, either primary or secondary, as a potential cause.

11. Are hormonal tests needed before surgery?

No. Hormonal tests are needed in only a minority of patients who have clinical signs of hormonal abnormalities. It is unnecessary to conduct the tests in everyone.

12. If the hormonal tests reveal any abnormality, then what should I do?

If the hormone analysis is abnormal, then you will need a thorough evaluation by an endocrinologist. However, in most cases, you will still need surgery to cure gynecomastia.

13. What is the procedure before I can undergo the surgery?

Before the surgery, you will need to get certain blood tests to assess your fitness to undergo the procedure. Once they are normal, then you can generally choose the anaesthesia you would prefer for the surgery. The procedure can be done under local anaesthesia (with or without intravenous supplementation) or general anaesthesia.

In local anaesthesia, the aesthetic injections are injected into the chest before the procedure is started. In general anaesthesia, you will be completely unaware of the whole process. Most surgeons and patients prefer general anaesthesia as it is much smoother in terms of surgery, recovery and pain.

14. How should I prepare for surgery?

If you are a smoker, you will be asked to stop smoking well in advance of surgery. Aspirin and certain anti-inflammatory drugs can cause increased bleeding, so you should avoid taking these medications for some time before surgery. Your surgeon will provide you with additional pre-operative instructions. Gynecomastia surgery is usually performed on an outpatient basis. If this is the case, be sure to arrange for someone to drive you home after surgery and to stay with you for at least the next day or two.

15. What happens during the day of the procedure?

On the day of the procedure, you will have to read, understand and sign a consent form for the procedure. The surgeon will do necessary markings on the chest skin, delineating the breast tissue along with the fat deposits to be tackled. He may point out any asymmetries and the scar location during the markings. Then, you will be started on a few injections through an intravenous cannula. Then, your chest and armpit hair are shaved (if not already done). In the operation theatre, you will be given certain injections along with oxygen for inhalation through a gas mask. Then, you will fall asleep and wake up only after the procedure is complete. When you wake up you will notice a dressing over your chest which will feel tight.

16. What is the surgical technique of gynecomastia correction?

The most common technique for gynecomastia correction is lipo-excision. It is a combination of liposuction (removal of fat) and gland excision (removal of breast gland). The liposuction is better done through the same site where the incision of excision is going to be. Some surgeons may use a small liposuction incision on the chest and may leave a small additional scar there.

Once the liposuction is done for the whole of the chest, excision is started. It is where the surgeon makes a half peri-areolar incision to remove the excess glandular tissue. During the removal of the gland, some surgeons leave about five to 20 percent of the gland behind so that the shape of the chest is much smoother as opposed to complete removal where the chest may look sunken. Some surgeons only use liposuction but, in most cases, this is a mistake unless it is pseudo gynecomastia (all fat content). Many unhappy patients come for re-do surgery following either only liposuction or only excision.

17. Which method of liposuction is used?

Like liposuction surgery, even in lipo-excision, the choice of the method depends on various factors like the area and quantity of fat to be removed, the associated side effects and recovery time, the surgeon's preference, cost, etc. Before surgery, it is important to decide on the method of liposuction after a detailed discussion on the pros and cons of each method. Check the chapter on liposuction Q and A for more details on the types of liposuction.

18. Will the breast gland that is left behind regrow?

The breast tissue does not grow after puberty. It can, however, increase slightly in size after the surgery in rare chromosomal anomalies and severe hormonal disturbances.

19. How painful is liposuction?

The pain factor depends primarily on the type of anaesthesia (local or general anaesthesia) and the extent of surgery. Most patients report minimal discomfort under local anaesthesia. Lipo-excision under general anaesthesia is painless as the individual is fully anesthetised.

20. If I have loose skin after the procedure, then what should I do?

This is a difficult and, often, a more complicated problem. The skin has a tremendous ability to contract, especially if a patient is young. In grade IIB and III gynecomastia, loose skin can sometimes persist. In such situations, the patient is reassessed after at least three months and the need for further skin tightening is discussed. It is however rare in most patients in early grades.

21. How will the recovery period progress?

The initial recovery period is three to seven days after your procedure. Total recovery time can vary from patient to patient. Most patients can expect to be fully healed by three to six weeks. The final results will, however, be obvious after three months. At this point, most or all of the bruising and swelling should have dissipated and the scars should have begun to shrink and fade. Sometimes, it may take as long as a year to completely heal to the point where the scars are almost no longer visible. For the first three to six weeks after surgery, it is necessary to avoid all strenuous activities, especially those involving the upper body such as lifting weights or intense workouts at the gym. Besides, patients are advised to wear a compression garment for six weeks post-operatively.

After the surgery, you will need to massage the operated area twice daily for at least three weeks. This helps the swelling to reduce faster and the skin to even out better. Also, the pressure garment is mandatory for proper reshaping of the chest. The following diagram depicts the general post-surgery protocol:

Your Daily Operated Site Care Schedule—To be followed in the morning and evening

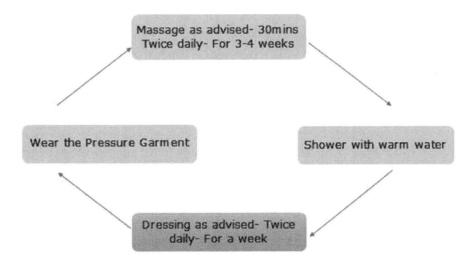

22. Are drains used after the procedure?

Some surgeons use drains. Drains help reduce swelling and promote better skin condition following your procedure. However, with newer and meticulous techniques, drains are not always mandatory.

23. What stitches are used after the procedure?

Most surgeons use dissolving stitches that fall off in two weeks, while others may prefer stitches that need to be removed after seven to ten days.

24. What are the psycho-social effects of gynecomastia and how are they affected by surgery?

Many studies and findings suggest that young men suffer emotional distress concerning gynecomastia. They feel socially isolated as they are unable to go out bare-chested during swimming or other activities. They also feel they cannot wear tight-fitting garments due to the chest bulge. Some suffer from depression and emotional distress, which is very often overlooked. Studies have assessed the physical and psycho-social aspects of the condition and how it changes after the gynecomastia is corrected. It is an accepted fact that gynecomastia surgery significantly improves the psycho-social outlook of such patients.

25. What are the complications after gynecomastia surgery?

The potential risks or complications associated with male breast reduction may include bleeding, infection, hematoma and delayed wound healing. The collection (seroma/hematoma), if less in quantity, will be absorbed by the body even without any intervention. If, however, the collection is large in quantity, an aspiration and compression will be needed. Delayed wound healing is especially seen in chronic smokers and hence they need to be advised to quit as early as possible.

26. Will there be any scarring with the surgery?

The incisions are normally made around the areola masking the appearance of scars especially because it is at the junction of darker areolar skin and the surrounding lighter skin of the chest. With the appropriate post-operative scar management, your male breast reduction scarring should be minimal.

Summary of Gynecomastia Surgery

Duration of procedure: 2-3 hours

Duration of hospital stay: 0-1 day

Need for follow-up: Once or twice

Stitch removal: Yes/No

Chapter 11

LIPOSUCTION Q AND A

This chapter has been added for relevant information about one of the most misunderstood procedures. Though it is used as a part of lipo-excision in gynecomastia correction; liposuction as a stand-alone procedure has many applications. Here are the basic pointers that will make you familiar with liposuction:

1. What is liposuction?

Liposuction is a surgical procedure performed to eliminate fat located in specific areas of the body. It is indicated for patients who have good skin elasticity. Liposuction objectively improves the body contour and outline. However, it should not be confused with a weight loss method. It is widely accepted more as a body contouring surgery.

2. How is liposuction done?

The liposuction begins with micro-incision (two to five millimetres wide) in the skin, through which fat is sucked out using special cannula and apparatus. Once the incision is done, the surgeon infiltrates fluid with various additives like adrenaline, sodium bicarbonate, hyaluronidase, etc. to soften up the fat. After waiting for the action of the infiltrate to set in, the surgeon then proceeds to remove the fat using a negative pressure vacuum device attached to long, narrow instruments called cannulas. The size of the cannulas can range from one to five millimetres in diameter. The size is chosen depending on the area to be treated, the size of fat in the location, etc. This process can last from 30 minutes to five hours depending on the area to be treated. The end point of liposuction is when adequate correction is achieved. The other important factor a surgeon is aware of is the safe limit of liposuction.

It is generally accepted that removing more than 15 litres of fat in a session of liposuction is unsafe. It leads to various electrolyte imbalances and considerable blood loss. So, the target is to remove well below the 15-litre limit.

3. Am I a Good Candidate for Liposuction Surgery?

A good candidate for liposuction is someone who has realistic expectations, is in reasonably good health and is likely to be happy with the results of liposuction. Although liposuction can often provide very substantial improvements, it is not always that liposuction results can be perfect. Following liposuction, the new body's shape is more or less permanent. If a patient does gain a moderate amount of weight after liposuction, then the figure will simply be a larger version of the new body shape. Fat cells that are removed by liposuction do not grow back.

It does not, however, mean that after the procedure the patient can forget about having a reasonable diet and exercise schedule. Though the amount of fat removed may never come back, it is, however, possible that the results obtained after the surgery may not last exactly how it had been immediately after recovery. The reason is that, though the fat cells may not multiply, they can increase in size to an extent if there is no adherence to a decent diet and exercise regimen. It is also important to bear in mind that a good candidate is someone who has stubborn areas of fat that cannot be eliminated with diet or exercise.

4. What is BMI and why is it important?

Body Mass Index (BMI) is a person's weight in kilograms divided by the square of height in metres. A high BMI can be an indicator of excess body fatness. BMI is used to screen for weight categories that may lead to health problems but it is not diagnostic of the body fatness or health of an individual. For adults (20 years old and older), BMI is interpreted using standard weight categories. These categories are the same for men and women of all body types and ages.

The standard weight status categories associated with BMI ranges for adults are shown in the following table.

BMI	Weight Category
Below 18.5	Underweight
18.5 – 24.9	Normal or Healthy Weight
25.0 – 29.9	Overweight
30.0 – 34.9	Moderately Obese
35.0– 39.9	Severely Obese
Above 40.0	Morbidly Obese/Very Severely Obese

5. Who is not a good candidate for liposuction?

The obvious bad candidates are those with unrealistic expectations. That, however, can be subjective and sometimes difficult to understand. Another clear method of identifying if someone is not suitable for the procedure is if the person is not inclined towards a healthy lifestyle and is looking for a short way out. People with stubborn pockets of fat even upon losing weight may now be candidates for liposuction.

People with a BMI over 30 should be careful while choosing liposuction, the main reason being that they may usually need multiple sittings of liposuction for a reasonable outcome. Someone with a BMI above 35 and with associated health problems like diabetes, arthritis or other metabolic diseases merits a bariatric surgery. The same holds for someone with a BMI over 40 even without the associated disorders.

6. What is bariatric surgery?

Bariatric surgery is a modality that provides a significant weight loss for morbidly obese patients, with resultant improvement in obesity-related disorders. Surgery for obesity should be considered as a treatment of last resort after dieting, exercise, psychotherapy, and drug treatments have failed.

7. Is liposuction safe?

This is probably the most important question that one needs to ask before jumping in. Liposuction is a relatively safe procedure. But there are risks and potential complications associated with any surgery and liposuction is no different. It is imperative to discuss long and hard about these with the surgeon.

Possible liposuction Risks are infection, extended healing time, allergic reaction to medication or anaesthesia, fat or blood clots (clots can migrate to the lungs and lead to death), excessive fluid loss (fluid loss can lead to shock and, in some cases, death), fluid accumulation/ Seroma (fluid must be drained), friction burns, scarring, numb skin, changes in skin pigmentation, damage to the skin or nerves and damage to vital organs.

Severe complications associated with liposuction are fortunately extremely rare but should be taken into consideration when deciding whether liposuction is right for you. These complications include adverse reactions to anaesthesia, cardiac arrest, cardiac arrhythmia, internal blood clots, excessive bleeding, severe drug interactions, allergic reactions to medication, permanent nerve damage, seizures and brain damage from anaesthesia.

The most common dangers of liposuction include risks associated with removing too much fat from targeted areas at once, as well as having too much liposuction performed in a single day. Excessive liposuction can cause problems including dents, lumps, and sagging skin. To minimise surgical complications and the side effects of overexposure to anaesthesia, when patients are looking to remove larger portions of fat, they should schedule multiple liposuction procedures at least several weeks apart.

8. How can you minimise the risks?

You can minimise your risk for severe complications by disclosing your entire medical history to your doctor and discussing all prescriptions and medications you take regularly. You and your surgeon should also make sure you are a good candidate for liposuction and fully understand what is involved in this procedure.

To maximise the success of liposuction surgery and minimise your risks, always follow your cosmetic surgeon's instructions for surgical preparation and post-operative care. If you smoke, your cosmetic surgeon will advise you to stop two weeks before and also following liposuction surgery. You may also choose another avenue for fat removal. There are non-surgical liposuction alternatives available to patients who are not good candidates for liposuction or simply prefer other methods.

9. What are the sequelae after liposuction?

Some sequel following liposuction is often referred to as 'temporary side effects.' In addition to the risks mentioned above, liposuction does cause some common side effects, which typically dissipate within a few weeks of the procedure and are hence sequelae.

Swelling: Liposuction will cause some swelling afterward, although some techniques cause less than others. During follow-up visits with a doctor, a patient needs to inform the doctor of any changes in the amount of post-liposuction swelling. Significant increases in swelling can be a warning sign of other complications. Swelling in the ankles and treated areas are common, along with a temporary lumpy appearance that will typically fade within six months. If the thighs are treated, inflammation of the veins may occur, but this should also go away after a few weeks.

Bruising: Another liposuction side effect is bruising. Treated areas may become discoloured and be tender to the touch, but they usually disappear after three to four weeks. Like swelling, the particular type of liposuction used can help mitigate any bruising that may occur. The status of the bruises should also be discussed with the doctor in post-surgery check-ups.

Discomfort: Following liposuction, patients often experience some soreness and tenderness in the treatment area. This can usually be controlled by pain medication. However, this discomfort is typically minimal and patients can return to work about two days after their procedures. If they experience severe discomfort or if the soreness gets worse after several days, patients should alert their doctors.

10. What is the duration of the surgery?

Most surgeries are between 45 minutes and two and a half hours, depending on the target area and method of liposuction.

11. How many areas can be done during liposuction in one sitting?

Usually, between three to four areas can safely be done with a single liposuction procedure. If additional areas are needed, they can be scheduled later.

12. What are the different types of liposuction?

There are several techniques that a surgeon can use to eliminate fat. At your consultation, the doctor will help you choose the right one for your needs. Liposuction procedures are many and are best chosen by an experienced surgeon.

MANUAL TECHNIQUES

Although manual liposuction does not utilise lasers, these treatments still use cutting-edge technology to minimise risks and provide stunning results. Manual options include:

Traditional Liposuction: In traditional liposuction, the surgeon uses a thin tube called a cannula, connected to a powerful suction pump or high suction syringes. After inserting the cannula through a small incision, the plastic surgeon helps break up the fat by manipulating the cannula and injecting fluid into the area. Although it does carry some risks, traditional liposuction is very effective in taking out fat and it is still one of the most popular forms of the procedure.

Tumescent Liposuction: Tumescent liposuction is similar to traditional liposuction but experts often hail its innovative use of medication and reduced risks for complications. During tumescent liposuction, the doctor will inject a special solution (a mixture of saline, local anaesthetic and adrenaline) into the layer of fat. The amount of fluid is usually three times the amount of fat being removed. The solution swells the fat cells, making them easier to isolate and remove. It also shrinks blood vessels and, because it contains local anaesthesia, it can help ease discomfort without the risks associated with general anaesthesia. Any minimal risks involve how much of the solution is injected, and how much lidocaine it contains.

Super-wet Liposuction: Super-wet liposuction is a variation of the tumescent technique that uses less fluid injection. The amount of fluid is usually equal to the amount of fat being removed. A general anaesthetic is required for this type of liposuction.

Ultrasonic Liposuction: This popular form of liposuction uses a specialised cannula that emits ultrasonic sound waves into the fat deposits to liquefy fat cells and make them easier to remove. By utilising ultrasound technology, the doctor can remove larger and denser fat deposits and he or she can tighten the surrounding skin. However, there is a small risk of burns and scarring due to the heat from the ultrasound waves.

LipoSelection®: This specialised form of liposuction, emulsifies fat cells with ultrasound and breaks them up even further with the

LipoSelection probe. The doctor can then easily remove the fat with liposuction tubes, leaving the surrounding blood vessels, nerves and other tissue virtually unaffected.

Power-Assisted Liposuction: By employing a cannula that has a vibrating tip, surgeons can break up fat cells for easier removal. Power-assisted liposuction also allows further fat removal, smaller incisions and reduced recovery time. This procedure is quite safe since the cannula can be moved with smaller, more exact movements. In some cases, however, patients may have looser skin than they desired.

TYPES OF LASER LIPOSUCTION

Advanced surgical lasers can loosen fat cells and make them easier to remove. Although they are typically more expensive than manual liposuction techniques, many patients feel that these procedures are worth the extra cost, since they typically enjoy less discomfort and a faster recovery time. Laser liposuction procedures include:

CoolLipo: This minimally invasive technique is designed for sensitive areas like the neck, jowls, arms and underneath the chin. CoolLipo also tightens skin with minimal bruising and utilises only local anaesthetic.

SlimLipo: SlimLipo lasers melt the fat cells before they are removed, reducing the discomfort and swelling associated with traditional liposuction. Some patients can even go to work the day after the procedure.

SmartLipo: This technique creates minimal scarring and is used for fine-tuning, removing only up to eight pounds of fat at a time. As with SlimLipo, patients can often return to work a day or two after their procedures.

13. Which method of liposuction should I choose?

The choice of the method depends on various factors like the area and quantity of fat to be removed, the associated side effects and recovery time, the surgeon's preference, cost, etc. Before surgery, it is important to decide on the method of liposuction after a detailed discussion on the pros and cons of each method.

14. When can I exercise?

You will be up and moving the day of your surgery. It is recommended that one should start a light physical activity as soon as possible the next day. Most patients return to their regular exercise routine between one to two weeks, although they may engage in mild exercise before that.

15. When can I see the results?

Final results usually take between one to four months but most patients see the beginning of results within one month. Usually, by three weeks much of the swelling is down and most patients are looking better than before the surgery and can wear a proper fitting dress.

16. Can I combine liposuction with other procedures?

In general, it is possible to combine other cosmetic procedures with liposuction. It is, however, important to take into consideration the extent of liposuction. If liposuction is a major one that may involve long surgical time or long recovery period it is not advisable to combine any other procedure. They can always be scheduled later.

17. What happens at my first consultation?

During the initial consultation, you may be asked to look in a mirror and point out exactly what you would like to see improved. This will help your plastic surgeon understand your expectations and determine whether they can realistically be achieved. A determination of the elasticity of the skin will also occur. Once this is over the surgeon will go over your surgical plan, ask any remaining questions and schedule your surgery and pre-op appointment.

18. What happens before surgery?

Once you have elected to move forward with surgery, a pre-op appointment will be scheduled anywhere from two weeks to ten days before your surgery date. This appointment will include blood tests, ultrasound scans, pre-op consents, pre and post-op instructions and garment measurements. You will also meet with your surgeon one more time so he can answer any remaining questions you may have.

19. What happens after surgery?

After liposuction, patients may feel nausea, grogginess and the sedate feeling that comes with general anaesthesia. You should be able to walk out of the surgery centre and be driven home by a companion or nurse to relax for the remainder of the day. You can usually return to work within two days. Physical exercise generally can be resumed three to seven days after liposuction. You will most likely come for a follow-up appointment within a week after surgery to check on incisions and make sure the healing process is going as planned. A long-term check-up is usually scheduled to check the final results.

20. How much fat is typically removed?

During liposuction, enough fat is removed to get a proportionate and natural result. It depends on your specific case and the areas being tackled. The goal is not to remove as much fat as possible, but rather to remove just the right amount in the right areas. It may be as little as half a litre, or it may be up to 15 litres.

21. What are the limitations of liposuction?

One thing that should be clear is not to use liposuction as a method for overall weight loss. It is solely a shaping/contouring procedure for areas where genetic fat deposits have proven to be resistant to diet and exercise. The best results from liposuction occur in body areas where there is a reasonable muscle tone, where the skin has a good elastic quality, and where fat is not overtly excessive. In cases where there is a significant loss of elasticity, proper cosmetic results may require a combination of both liposuction and surgical skin tightening to remove the excessive loose tissue. For example: Tummy Tuck.

22. What is the most amount of fat that can be removed?

The safe limit for one surgery is less than 15 litres. But more importantly, it is not the amount of fat that limits the surgery but how many areas can be safely done during a single surgery taking into consideration various patient factors.

23. At what age can a patient have liposuction performed?

As long as all physical criteria are met for liposuction candidacy, liposuction can technically be performed on anyone 15 to 78 years old. However, skin elasticity is a primary consideration when performing liposuction. As one's age advances, skin elasticity gets weaker and weaker. If the surgeon feels the skin's elasticity is poor, he may recommend other procedures to reach the cosmetic goals.

24. How painful is liposuction?

The pain factor depends primarily on the type of anaesthesia (local or general anaesthesia) and the extent of surgery. Most patients report minimal discomfort during liposuction under local anaesthesia. The first step of such a procedure is injection of local anaesthetic, which takes about 15 to 30 minutes to set in. During this time, patients report a mild pinching sensation. Once the local anaesthetic has taken root, patients report no pain at all.

Liposuction under general anaesthesia is painless as the individual is fully anesthetised.

25. What happens on the Day of Liposuction Surgery?

Medications are administered for your comfort during the surgical procedure. Frequently, local anaesthesia and intravenous sedation are used for patients undergoing liposuction surgery, although general or spinal anaesthesia may be desirable in some instances. For your safety during the operation, various monitors are used to check your heart, blood pressure, pulse and the amount of oxygen circulating in your blood.

When surgery is completed, you will be taken into a recovery area where you will continue to be closely monitored. You will most likely be wearing a compression garment or a tight dressing, usually used to help "shrink" the skin. Concerning post-operative pain, many patients state that the area feels sore as if they underwent a vigorous workout. You probably will be permitted to go home after a short period of observation, although some patients may stay overnight in the hospital or surgical facility.

26. Is liposuction better before or after pregnancy?

Because liposuction works best on areas of good skin tone, it is generally better to have it done before pregnancy. However, each case is unique and the surgeon can recommend which procedure will best suit your needs, before or after pregnancy. It also depends on the area that needs liposuction and the skin tone.

27. Will I have loose skin after liposuction?

You will not have loose skin following liposuction if your skin tone is good to begin with. When liposuction is done properly, the skin re-drapes and retracts to conform to the underlying tissue. Skin elasticity is vital to a good procedure. For this reason, the surgeon will perform a thorough examination to determine your skin elasticity. If he finds it may not support the new contours following liposuction, he may recommend other treatments.

28. What happens if I gain weight after liposuction?

When liposuction is performed correctly, the contours of the body should be permanently improved. In other words, if you gain weight, your new contours and proportions should remain more or less the same as they were after liposuction. Weight gain will simply make these contours a little less visible. If you then lose the weight again, your contours should resume their post-liposuction size and shape.

29. How are the post-liposuction scars?

Each incision is usually between one to five millimetres in length. This is usually small enough to prevent the need for stitches following surgery. Multiple incisions may be needed to adequately treat the target treatment areas. However, these are usually well-hidden and heal without incident. In a rare case that an incision becomes unsightly, many techniques are available to help reduce their appearance.

30. Can I go home on the same day?

Yes, you go can home very shortly after surgery. However, it is necessary to have a friend or family member drive you. It is recommended that you don't drive for the first 24 hours after surgery. It is also recommended that you have a companion with you for the first several hours after surgery. Most liposuctions are day care procedures but, when done extensively, there may be a need for an extended admission.

31. Is it normal to be anxious before having liposuction surgery?

Yes. Almost everyone has some degree of anxiety before having a surgical procedure, including liposuction. Some people have more anxious than others. You may be administered medications to lower your stress levels.

32. How does abdominal liposuction differ from a 'Tummy Tuck'?

A tummy tuck (abdominoplasty) is a more major surgical procedure requiring general or spinal anaesthesia and involves liposuction and excision to remove fat, plus removal of a large area of skin. In many patients (but not all), liposuction of the abdomen can often provide equivalent or better results than a tummy tuck. Because liposuction is safer and causes less scarring compared to tummy tucks, abdominal liposuction is now far more common than are tummy tucks. However, Tummy Tuck is definitely indicated in people with excess loose skin especially following pregnancy.

33. What about touch-ups?

With liposuction in general, there is a chance for the requirement of revisions. However, the requirement depends on the areas that were operated upon, surgical expertise, etc.

34. What are the chances of irregularities, dimples, or asymmetry occurring after liposuction?

The chance of defects or flaws after liposuction when done by an experienced surgeon is very low. He/she would everything in his power to achieve a smooth, natural result and a happy patient. If the surgeon feels your chances of irregularities are high due to poor skin elasticity or skin tone, he/she should discuss this with you extensively and may recommend another treatment option.

35. What are the post-procedure instructions?

Following the procedure, the patient is prescribed antibiotics, pain killers, antacids, medication to reduce swelling and nausea. But the main post-surgical care involves the use of compression garment and massage of the operated area. The patient is also prescribed antiseptic ointments to be applied to the incisions.

36. How long do I need to wear a compression garment?

Patients are generally asked to wear the compression garment for at least six weeks full-time after surgery. The duration again depends on the skin laxity, size of the gland and other factors.

37. How does massage help after liposuction?

The benefits of massage after liposuction lack consensus. However, it is better to start massage once the pain is tolerable after the procedure. It should be done using a copious amount of moisturiser/oil and in circular fashions with moderate pressure. Lymphatic massage may also be advised in some cases. Occasionally, some people feel comfortable getting them done by a therapist. The massage also should be continued for at least three weeks and done thrice daily.

38. When can I fly?

In most cases, you may fly two days after the surgery as long as you can walk around every hour while on the plane.

39. How much does liposuction cost?

Many factors are taken into account when quoting liposuction costs. The factors include—degree of difficulty, amount of fat to be removed, number of areas to be treated, operating room fees, anaesthesiologist fees, type of liposuction, etc.

Each of these factors will be assessed before your procedure and you will be given a number. The number may change slightly through the course of the procedure depending on your stay and recovery course.

40. Does insurance cover liposuction?

Summary of Gynecomastia Surgery

Duration of procedure: 2-3 hours

Duration of hospital stay: 0-1 day

Need for follow-up: Once or twice

Stitch removal: Yes/No

No, because it is a purely cosmetic procedure.

"*Do not go gentle into that good night,*

Old age should burn and rave at close of day;

Rage, rage against the dying of the light.

Though wise men at their end know dark is right,

Because their words had forked no lightning they

Do not go gentle into that good night.

Good men, the last wave by, crying how bright

Their frail deeds might have danced in a green bay,

Rage, rage against the dying of the light.

Wild men who caught and sang the sun in flight,

And learn, too late, they grieved it on its way,

Do not go gentle into that good night.

Grave men, near death, who see with blinding sight

Blind eyes could blaze like meteors and be gay,

Rage, rage against the dying of the light.

And you, my father, there on the sad height,

Curse, bless, me now with your fierce tears, I pray.

Do not go gentle into that good night.

Rage, rage against the dying of the light."

– Dylan Thomas

– Made famous after it featured in the movie 'Interstellar.'

DR SREEKAR'S WEBSITES AND SOCIAL MEDIA PLATFORMS

1. Facebook

https://www.facebook.com/drsreekarh/

2. Instagram:

https://www.instagram.com/dr.sreekar.harinatha/

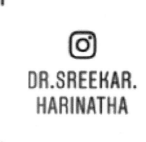

3. Dedicated website for gynecomastia info

www.gynecomastiabangalore.com

4. Cosmetic surgery website

www.conturacosmetic.com

NOTES

Printed in Great Britain
by Amazon

78218944R00105